LOOKING PRETTY,
FEELING FINE

LOOKING PRETTY, FEELING FINE

❧ ❧

Marjabelle Young Stewart

Illustrations by Durell Godfrey

David McKay Company, Inc.

NEW YORK

Library of Congress Cataloging in Publication Data

Stewart, Marjabelle Young.
  Looking pretty, feeling fine.
  Includes Index

  SUMMARY: A teenage girls' guide to such topics as grooming, nutrition, job hunting, and dating.
    1. Adolescent girls—Health and hygiene. 2. Beauty, Personal. 3. Adolescent girls—Conduct of life. [1. Grooming. 2. Health. 3. Beauty, Personal. 4. Dating (Social customs)] I. Godfrey, Durell. II. Title.
RA778.S82   646.7   79-13619
ISBN 0-679-51178-4

1 2 3 4 5 6 7 8 9 10

Manufactured in the United States of America

This book is lovingly dedicated
To Erin Marjabelle Anderson
AND
Margaret Eve Louise Caruso

ACKNOWLEDGMENTS

My thanks and appreciation beyond words to Marian Faux for her vast professional competence and excellent judgment. Without her, quite literally, this book would not have been possible.

To Cindy Nelson, my immediate editor for her unfailing encouragement and generosity, which, along with her exacting publishing standards, are reflected throughout the staff of the David McKay Company.

My particular gratitude and admiration to my agent, Dominick Abel, for his understanding and kindness in helping me past the scores of emergencies, big and little, that marked my development as an author.

CONTENTS

FOREWORD

⨯§ Almost every young girl dreams of being beautiful, but few are sure how to achieve beauty. Must you begin with flawless features? Must you imitate the major fashion models? And what if you simply can't do this because you are too short or too tall, or too anything else? Can an average-looking teen become beautiful, or must you be born that way? And, to get down to the nitty-gritty of the issue, why do all the boys seem to like that one girl, whom you don't find *that* pretty?

The reason that most teens have trouble sorting out what beauty means is that they have not yet had time to develop their own style—the kind that brings out their own personal beauty.

Most models and other people you especially admire for looking pulled-together or even beautiful are self-made, for the fact is that few of us are born with features that everyone agrees are beautiful.

So if you aren't born with natural, stunning good looks, how can you achieve the aura of having beauty, as so many models and other "beauties" of our time do? The answer is in two parts. First, you can learn all there is to know about grooming and caring for yourself so that you always look your best. This is the foundation. Second, you can work to develop the self-assurance that makes others believe you are attractive.

The larger part of this book is devoted to physical grooming —looking your best all the time. This is because being well-groomed is merely a matter of learning. You need, first, to pick up the basics, plus a few tricks of the modeling trade— and, gradually, you will find that you are quite capable of making the most of your looks.

The second part of the book is devoted to getting along with others—making your friends feel good about themselves, making a good impression at school, attracting boys. The chapters that deal with these subjects contain ideas and hints to help you feel more confident, but they also contain a little bit of philosophy about how you might want to look at life. When you look your best and feel your best, it is easier to relate to others. And relating to others is mostly a matter of caring and thinking about others' needs, wishes, and wants. It is about consideration. And this comes from having a good feeling about yourself and about your relationships. We do offer some hints and suggestions to help you get started and to get you over any initial shyness, but you will find that the more you practice your social skills, the easier it will be to relate to other people.

Does this all sound simple? It *is* fairly easy, although becoming the person you want to be does take time and effort. Mostly, though, being popular involves doing everything you can to enhance your looks and then forgetting about them while you go out and make others feel good. This is the secret of feeling and being attractive.

In recent years, teenage girls and boys have begun to look more and more alike. They wear the same clothes. They may have the same haircut. They are often active in the same sports. Teen girls wear less makeup and devote less time to personal grooming than they did ten or twenty years ago. And in many ways, this is good. Young skin does not need a lot of makeup. A healthy body that is achieved by playing the same sports that boys play is far better than one kept in shape with a set of exercises. We are hardly suggesting that today's teens drop the very things that are so good for them. But we do feel that it is important to be aware of your looks, how to develop your own personal style, and how to dress well on those occasions when you choose to shed your jeans. Or for that matter, how to dress well in jeans. To emerge as a self-confident young woman, you need to learn what works for you.

Not everything in this book will appeal to every reader. You may, at age sixteen, already have enough of a sense of what you are all about to know that eye makeup is not for you. That is wonderful. But you also need to know what the possibilities are—how you can shape yourself and improve your looks with grooming and makeup techniques if you want to. You need to know how to diet in a healthy way when you have gained too many extra pounds. You need to know what exercise program is right for you if you aren't inclined to play basketball with the boys.

You should pick and choose the things in this book that are helpful to you. This is, I hope, a book that will help you develop lifelong habits of good grooming—which, in turn, will increase your self-confidence. This is the book that will help your personal style—whatever it may be—emerge.

—*Marjabelle Young Stewart*
JANUARY 1979

1

TAKING STOCK

&§ Self-confidence stems from an appreciation of your own worth—from knowing that you always look your best and that you are fun to be around. It is not to be confused with an obsessive concern about yourself or with vanity, for these are different things. Learning to make the best of your looks, for example, does not require that you spend all your free time thinking about them. Rather, it requires that you learn certain basics of good grooming and then stick with them, leaving your mind free for other matters.

You can also learn how to get along with others, how to be a good friend to another girl, and how to make boys like you and enjoy your company. You can learn the ease of displaying good manners that will make you popular with everyone you meet. Knowing all these things helps you to have and maintain self-confidence. This book shows you how to make the most of your looks, but it also talks a lot about making the most of your personality, about projecting yourself in a pleasing way.

Most of us at one time or another have some self-doubts. We think people don't like us. We don't have a best friend. We weren't chosen to be student council representative. We think our noses are too big, our breasts are too small—and nothing we put on seems to look exactly right. Some of this may be true. You have to be a good friend to have a good friend. You may also have a physical trait that needs some self-improvement. But mostly, the things that appear to be wrong with us are not unfixable. And this book tells you how to go about fixing those things—how to strengthen your weak areas and how to bring out your strengths.

So many factors enter into how one feels about oneself that it is difficult to help another person analyze how much or how little self-confidence she may have. The two questionnaires below, one of which deals with your feelings and the other with your looks, may help you organize your feelings about yourself. These are "thinking" questions. There are no right or wrong answers; we hope that these questions will mostly start you thinking more about how and why you feel the way you do. If you answer yes to six or more of the questions on each questionnaire, you feel pretty good about yourself. If you answer no to six or more questions—or even to enough questions to make you feel uncomfortable—then you might want to think about ways to make yourself feel better. You might want to plan your wardrobe more carefully, go on a diet, get more regular exercise—whatever you need, go out and do it for yourself. The guidance you need to embark on these new activities is all right here in this book.

As a final suggestion, try keeping a diary of your progress. You could begin the diary by writing down a private discussion with yourself over the questions to which you answered no. If you do not like the shape of your face, or you do not have a best friend, ask yourself why. Then ask yourself what you could be doing about this. And then work out a plan for self-improvement. Report to yourself on your progress in the diary.

Feeling Fine Questionnaire

1. Do you participate in as many school activities as you would like to?

2. Do you participate in at least one activity because it involves a special interest of yours?

3. Are you able to be friends with boys you do not date?

4. Do you rank having a boyfriend as being *no more important* and *no less important* than doing well in school, having a good time with your friends, and spending your free time in a pleasant, productive way?

5. Do you have a best girlfriend?

6. If one friend were unavailable to help you when you wanted to talk over a problem, do you have one or two other good friends you could call upon?

7. Do you genuinely feel sorry for a friend when she has had some bad luck or misfortune?

8. Do you go out, either with your friends or with a boyfriend, as often as you would like to?

9. Do you respect your parents' wishes fairly often, about 70 percent of the time, for example? (A little self-assertion is part of being a teen.)

10. Is at least one teacher a special friend to you? Would he or she notice if you underwent a serious mood change, changed friends, or suddenly gained or lost a lot of weight?

11. If you were really bothered by a problem, would you feel free to talk to a professional, i.e. a school counselor or a therapist?

12. Do you have several important goals or achievements that you are seeking in the future, i.e. a college you hope to be admitted to, a part-time job you really want, a club you hope to join?

Looking Pretty Questionnaire

1. Do you mostly like your body, that is, are you comfortable with it? Do you feel that your weight and shape, if not perfect, are quite acceptable?

2. Do you like the shape of at least one of your features to

the point where you think it balances out another, not-so-good feature?

3. Do you like the shape of your face?

4. Do you get at least five hours of exercise every week?

5. Do you maintain a fairly regular grooming routine?

6. Do you visit a dentist and eye doctor regularly?

7. Do you keep your closets and drawers fairly neat and well-organized?

8. Do you sometimes pull out all your clothes and study them to think of new ways to combine them and of new clothes and accessories that would enhance what you already own?

10. Do you think about changing something about yourself (your hair, the way you dress, how much exercise you get) and then do it?

11. Do you feel pretty self-confident about your looks most of the time? (Everyone has some bad days.)

Answering these questions and then writing out how you feel and what you can do to improve yourself should prepare you to embark on a minor or major self-improvement program. And all the tools you need to do this are in the chapters that follow. Good luck!

2

MAKEUP FOR TEENS

❧ Undoubtedly, one of the first signs of growing up is the urge to start wearing makeup. Most girls want to start when their peers do, and this is usually around age twelve or thirteen. Of course, at this age you probably won't want to wear much makeup—perhaps a little baby powder and lip gloss—and you should not feel any pressure to wear makeup at all if you are not comfortable doing so.

Makeup is fun. It's very much like painting a picture. Makeup is also easily overdone, especially by young teens. Some girls think that wearing a lot of makeup makes them look older than they are. It does, but in a most unflattering way. In this book, you will learn how to wear makeup that is right for your age.

Few things are sadder or sillier than a teenager with heavy black-rimmed eyes, garish eye shadow, and too much rouge. Going light on makeup, however, does not mean wearing no makeup. There are several reasons to wear it, but the two most important are that 1) none of us is perfect, and makeup helps to hide little flaws—and 2) makeup is just too much fun not to try your hand at it.

Become a Good Consumer

If you are just beginning to wear makeup, you will have a lot to learn about it: what you will need, what colors look best on you, what is "in" right now, and which makeups are the best buys.

As with anything else you buy today, it pays to be a good consumer when shopping for makeup. Learn to read labels carefully. Some products still contain certain ingredients that are dangerous. Do not buy any makeup that contains mercury, lead, or bismuth of salts, for example. Magazines and newspapers provide a constant flow of information about how healthful various ingredients are in cosmetics—read these carefully and you will be a wiser consumer.

You should also learn to pay attention to the sizes of cosmetics containers. Some cheap mascaras, for example, are really more expensive than the higher-priced ones, because the former contain so much less mascara. Whenever you are weighing the cost of an item, also consider its size.

A Word about Cleanliness

Before you start learning how to choose and apply makeup, you need to appreciate how important cleanliness is. Even people who scrupulously wash their faces twice a day often do not think about using an eye shadow applicator over and over without washing it or using a new one. Yet you must learn to be as clean as possible about everything that touches your skin. Don't use the same tissue over and over again. Learn to use two or three cotton balls instead of one miserly one. Foam rubber sponges for applying makeup base and foam rubber applicators for eye shadows can be purchased in any dime store. Learn to toss out old ones the minute they look used—or before. These items—all of which help to keep your skin clean—are among the cheapest beauty aids you will ever buy.

6

Following Fashion Versus Your Own Style

Finding the cosmetics that look wonderful on you takes a little experimenting. Makeup should be keyed to your coloring. Blondes usually look best in light, pastel colors. Brunettes or persons with brown hair can wear brighter colors. Redheads can, too, although they need to be careful not to overdo the color; when you've got red or auburn hair, you've got a head start in the color department.

Makeup styles change frequently, too. A few years ago, false eyelashes and heavy eyeliner were part of every fashionable woman's makeup; today, they are rarely worn. In recent years, a whole new cosmetic color family—brown—has been introduced in makeup. The browns and beiges are often especially flattering to teens. A good way to see what makeup is "in" is to look at fashion magazines, which report on makeup in every issue. But beware of following fashion too closely. The best look for most teens is a healthy, natural one—and that's not always the look that's in style at the moment. While it's fun to follow the new trends in makeup, you should always do so with an eye to maintaining a natural look.

Magazines often play up very sophisticated makeups. They may talk about toners that you wear under a base to subtly change the color of your skin, or they may describe a complicated method for changing the shape of your face with shadowing. This kind of makeup is too sophisticated for most people, let alone a young woman. Anyway, these techniques are usually used only by models on a regular basis—the rest of us content ourselves with a ten-minute makeup first thing in the morning.

In makeup, as with clothes, you should always stick to what looks best on you rather than the fashion of the moment. This is the sign of a truly chic woman, and no teen is ever too young to start looking chic.

Buying Makeup

Before you can start applying makeup, you must go out and buy some basic cosmetics. Since you will still be experimenting to find your best colors and the kinds of products that are best for you, you might want to haunt dime stores and drugstores, which carry fairly inexpensive lines of makeup. There is little difference in the content of most cosmetics—generally you pay more money for fancy packaging and a big name—so dime store makeup is perfectly alright to start out with. Here is a basic list of the makeup you will need to start with and the tools required to put it on correctly.

Basic Beginner's Cosmetics
base (sometimes called
   foundation)
lipstick
lip balm or other cream for
   dry lips
mascara
powder—either baby
   powder or a translucent
   kind
cheek coloring—blusher,
   rouge

Beginner's Tools
tweezers
mirror
facial tissues
brushes—for eyebrows, lips,
   and blusher

As you become more involved with makeup, there are other items you may want to add.

Special Cosmetics
   eye shadows
   eyeliners
   eyebrow pencil or shadow
   coverup
   under-makeup moisturizer
   variety of lipsticks
   special powder, eye shadow, and blusher for evening wear

As you invest in these makeup items, you will also want to acquire whatever is needed to use them—brushes, foam rubber applicators, or sponges.

Applying Makeup

Always start with immaculate skin. Once you have applied makeup, never put on more. This is asking for trouble, especially with a teenage skin. Tie a scarf or ribbon around your hair to pull it back off your face before you begin to apply makeup.

You should apply makeup in a good strong light. Some articles and books on makeup advise you to apply it according to the kind of light you will be in. That is, if you plan to be under fluorescent light—what many schools have—then you should make up in fluorescent light, or at least learn to apply makeup to compensate for the drained tone that skin takes on under this light. This is all well and good, except that few of us have makeup mirrors or home lighting sophisticated enough to duplicate all the various kinds of light we will encounter during the course of a day. Even if your school has fluorescent lights, you will still walk out into the bright sun after school and during lunch—and then your makeup will be all wrong, because bright sun requires very subtle, discreet makeup. Are you thinking that this is a no-win situation? You are right, and the best way to come out ahead is to develop a makeup routine that suits you and stick to it, regardless of the kind of light you will be in.

Actually, the only times you may want to vary your makeup routine are when you are participating in sports activities and when you are going out for a very special evening. For sports, most teens and grown women wear less makeup. Sweat shining through makeup is never attractive, so if you are planning an afternoon of tennis, sailing, or swimming, you will probably want to wear little, if any, makeup. For big evenings it is fun to wear special makeup—perhaps a pearlized powder or a shimmery eye shadow. Such glitter, however, is best saved only for these special events. Most of us just look like a jaded Tinkerbell when we start glittering too much during the daylight hours.

Applying Foundation

The first cosmetic you will apply is a foundation, also called a makeup base. (Some young women, who have already developed a tendency toward dry skin, may also need an under-makeup lotion. This is discussed more in Chapter 3, on skin care.)

There are basically two kinds of makeup base: water-based and oil-based. The water-based kind is best for most young skins, and oil-based foundations are best for dry skins, which few teens have. Foundations also come in several forms: cream, liquid, and cake. Even among these forms, there are variations. Some makeup companies make a light creamy base that looks as if it has been whipped; others make a heavy pancake makeup base. Most teens look best in a light liquid or cream base. Ask a salesperson to help you choose the best form for you.

A makeup base should match the color of your skin as closely as possible. You may want to vary a shade or two from your skin as a means of correcting a skin tone you are not crazy about, but this is something to be done very carefully. A sallow skin, for example, can be enlivened with a rosy-toned base, and a tan skin can be enhanced with a bronze-toned makeup base. Very fair skins usually take an ivory or slightly rosy makeup base. Black skin comes in a wide variety of shades, and since in recent years makeup companies have begun to cater to black skins, finding a shade to match your skin should not be difficult. If you have very dark skin and have trouble finding a good match, go to a shade darker rather than lighter.

To apply base, dab a few dots of it on your forehead, nose, cheeks, and chin. Now—using a sponge or your fingertips—blend it in with upward motions. Be careful not to get it in your hair, and do not apply to your neck. As a finishing touch, smooth it downward, the way the tiny hairs on your face grow. Apply carefully to your eyelids if you are planning to add eye shadow.

Many women of all ages tend to wear too much makeup base. You should never look as if you are wearing base, and it certainly should not form a mask one or two shades darker than your neck. A good way to be sure you have not overdone the base is to look carefully at your face and neck in a mirror held near a sunlit window. Your makeup should not show.

Applying Rouge

Once you have applied the base, it's time to apply rouge. Most of us need a little extra color on our cheeks, but if you happen to be blessed with naturally rosy cheeks, by all means skip this step. Rouges come in powder form (called blusher), liquid, and cream.

Liquids and creams take a lot of skill to apply, and for that reason most teens elect to use a powder rouge. Select a blusher to go with your skin tones. If you are blue-eyed and have light hair, a light-colored pink or peach or a light tawny brown will be right for you; brunettes and redheads may need a slightly stronger color. Also consider what outfit you will be wearing and what shade of lipstick you will use. A peach-colored blusher should not be worn with a pink lipstick and vice versa. The brown shades of makeup are very useful because you can wear them with more colors. With a light brown blusher, you probably won't have to worry about what color outfit or lipstick you are wearing, as it will blend in nicely.

Blusher should be applied with an upward motion to the outer edges of your cheeks. Do not apply it too close to your eyes or your nose, or you will look like a clown.

Sometimes the brush that comes with a blusher is hard to use; if this happens with the brand you buy, invest in a nice soft 1- to 1½-inch makeup or artist's brush and use that to apply your blusher.

11

Using Blusher to Contour

Now you are about to learn a model's trick—how to shape your face. Just remember that a little of this technique goes a long way.

The advantage of contouring is that by simply applying a little blusher to some strategic spots on your face, you can appear to change its shape. You can *minimize only,* though. A too-long nose will not vanish, nor will a round face suddenly become a perfect oval. Here, however, are some simple and effective ways to alter the appearance of your face shape, using a brown-toned blusher:

Face too long:
    apply blusher to center of cheeks

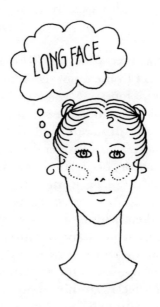

Face too square:
   apply along jawline as shown

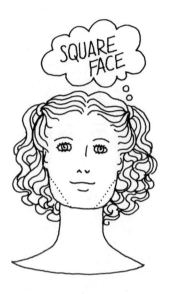

Face too round:
   apply downward in roundest area

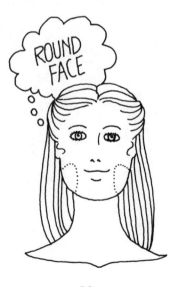

Nose too long
  apply a dab of blusher under its tip

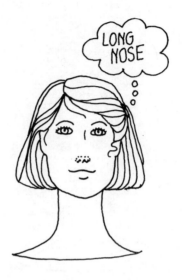

Nose too wide:
  apply blusher along both sides in narrow strips

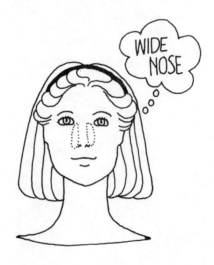

Chin too pointed:
  apply a small area of blusher on chin

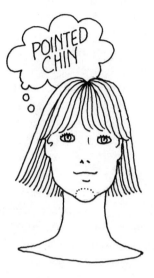

Pretty Eyes

After you have used base and blusher, you will need little more than a light coating of mascara, some eye shadow, and possibly a finishing dab of powder on your nose. The fashion magazines often carry articles on how to change the shape of your eyes through the use of eye shadow—this is, however, a touch too much makeup for most teens to carry off well. But before you toss this book aside and go out to buy three eye shadows to change the shape of your eyes, it's best to know that the shape of your eyes can't be drastically changed anyway. So for what it's worth, you're better off wearing very light touches of eye makeup rather than fancy three-tone jobs. (Later in this chapter, we'll show you how to apply eye shadow a little more elaborately for big party nights.)

Before you apply eye makeup, take a good look at your eyebrows, since they can overpower a lovely set of eyes if they are too heavy. Plucking eyebrows is mostly a job for professionals, and the natural look in eyebrows is in style today anyway. But if you think your eyebrows are excessively heavy, see if you can get your parents' permission to have them plucked or waxed by an expert working in a top beauty salon. After that, you will only need to pluck stray hairs from below and between your brows. Pluck in the direction the hairs grow, and never pluck from the top of your brows—for one thing, it hurts; for another, it is too easy to ruin the line of your brow.

Sparse eyebrows are another matter entirely, and if you think yours are too thin, this can be changed with the discreet application of an eyebrow powder or pencil. Try both kinds and see which works best for you. Buy a shade lighter than your eyebrows, and apply with very light, short strokes. No one should ever be able to tell that you have added color to fill in your brows.

Some teens also choose to wear a little eye shadow during the day. This is okay if you choose a quiet, soft color, and if you don't overdo it. Eye shadows come in cream, pencil, and powder form. Powder is probably the easiest to apply and looks the lightest. Stick to light shades; smoky or dark eye shadows will only make you look unhealthy, not sophisticated. Pearlized eye shadows are best saved for evening wear—what may look okay under the bathroom lights will look garish in bright sunlight.

Somewhat surprisingly, you should not match your eye shadow to your eye color. Blue eyes look best in grays, lavender, pale greens, and beiges; brown eyes in beiges, brown or copper shades, and soft greens; hazel eyes are played up by pale greens. Eye shadow, as the illustration indicates, can be applied in three areas: in the crease of your eye, on the lid, and right below the brow.

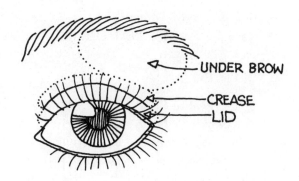

For daytime wear, few teens look good with eye shadow applied to all three areas. Most teens only wear a little in the crease or on the eyelid, depending upon what most flatters the eye shape. Also, do not ring your entire eye with shadow and do not apply a dark, heavy line in the crease of your eye. Wear just the merest hint of a shadow, wherever you decide to wear it.

Mascara is the final touch to your eyes. It, too, comes in several forms: liquid, cake, and in a tube, and the tube is probably easiest to use. Never wear black mascara, even if you have black hair—choose a dark brown shade if you have dark hair and a light brown if you have light-colored hair. Apply the mascara carefully, starting at the base of your lashes and moving to the tips. When applying it, hold your face up so your eyes are partially closed—this way you will get the mascara on your lashes and not your cheeks.

Let the mascara dry for a few minutes before you get dressed, and always check before you leave the house to be sure your mascara has not smeared.

Along with mascara comes the question of false eyelashes, eyelash curlers, and eyeliner. False eyelashes have really fallen out of style, and they look heavy anyway, so you may want to cross them off your list of possible beauty aids. Eyelash curlers are a necessity if you happen to be blessed with extravagantly long eyelashes and you wear glasses—curling them keeps them from hitting against the glasses (we should all be this lucky). Even if you don't have this "problem," you may still want to use an eyelash curler. It can be purchased in any dime store for a few dollars. Before you put on mascara, place the two rubber-lined metal pieces onto your lashes and clamp down for about fifteen seconds. Don't overcurl—it looks too obvious during the few hours it takes for your lashes to relax.

Eyeliner, currently not very popular, comes and goes with the times, and you may or may not want to use it, depending upon the shape of your eyes and the look you want to achieve. Eyeliner comes in pencil, liquid, and cake form. The pencil form—a brown shade is best—gives the softest look. Apply eyeliner as close to your lashes as you possibly can in a super-thin line, stopping where your lashes stop. You may want to smear it a little for an even softer look.

Lipsticks and How to Use Them

Actually, the first question you should ask yourself about lipstick is whether or not you even want to use it. A no-lipstick look has been popular for several years now, and few people can carry off this look better than a teenager. Instead of lipstick, you may want to use a lip gloss that adds shine and no color.

If you choose to use a lipstick with color, though, find one that goes well with your skin tone, your outfit, and your blusher. In other words, do not wear a peach lipstick with a pink outfit or a red lipstick with a peach blusher. Wearing makeup in the brown tones helps to solve this problem, as the browns tend to go with most skin tones and most clothing colors.

Apply lipstick on top of your makeup base. Lipstick should only be applied where you have lips, unless you are going to a party dressed as a 1940s movie star (that's the last time it was popular to reshape your lips in an obvious way). Lipstick also looks neater and wears better when applied with a lip brush.

To apply lipstick this way, first use a circular motion to put lipstick on the brush from the tube or container, working the brush into a fine point. Then carefully use the brush to outline your lips. Fill in with more lipstick applied to the brush or directly from the tube. Over this you can apply lip gloss if you want to.

Lipsticks come in a variety of colors and textures. Experiment to find the ones that are the best colors for you and that also seem to feel good on your skin.

The best lipstick colors for teens are light peaches, pinks, and browns. Brunettes and people with black skin look great in red tones, but these can sometimes be harsh, so be careful about selecting one of these shades.

The Finishing Touches

To set your makeup, you may want to apply a little face powder—baby powder or translucent powder works and looks best on young skins. If you have really good skin and do not live in a heavily polluted area, you can probably skip the makeup base and just use a light dusting of powder on your skin. The purpose of powder is to take away the shine on excessively shiny skin. Remember, however, that a little shine looks healthy—don't apply powder so heavily that you take it all away. Translucent powder works especially well on black skins.

Another way to set your makeup is to press a wet washcloth against it very lightly or mist it. Either of these techniques will help keep your makeup fresh-looking for hours.

Special Makeup Tips for Special Problems

PROBLEM: The senior prom is coming up in two weeks and I'm planning to wear a white dress. I think I will need some special makeup touches, but I'm not sure what will work and what won't.

ANSWER: Making up for special evenings is fun. It means you can apply your blusher with a little heavier hand, on the assumption that you will not be under bright lights. You can also apply a little more eye makeup. This might be the time to try eyeliner (assuming you have practiced to the point of perfection before the dance) or a sparkling pastel eye shadow. Ditto a pearlized blusher—this is a time to shine and sparkle.

PROBLEM: I have acne and my dermatologist has told me I can't wear any makeup at all. What can I do?

ANSWER: Follow your doctor's advice—except you might wear a makeup to cover your blemishes for special occasions. Just be very careful to wash off all traces before you go to bed. Wearing heavy makeup to cover blemishes—a perfectly normal tendency—will only make the condition worse in the long run.

PROBLEM: I have freckles, especially in the summer, and I think they're ugly. What creams will work to bleach them?

ANSWER: Rethink freckles, if you can. Most people think they're cute, and many a pale-skinned woman has been thankful for the added touch of color they give her during the winter months. If you want to avoid getting freckles, stay out of the sun. If you want to lessen freckles, try a makeup base to even the tone of your skin. Commercial creams that promise to remove freckles do not work, and some contain products such as mercury and lead that are actually harmful to your skin.

PROBLEM: I don't have blemishes anymore, but I still have some scars. What can I do to cover these?

ANSWER: Acne scars can be covered by using a special cosmetic designed for this purpose. Ask a salesperson at your favorite cosmetic counter to recommend something that will hide scars. Apply the undercover before you put on your base.

PROBLEM: I have a mole—a birthmark, I guess—on my cheek. Can I use a makeup to cover it?

ANSWER: Most makeups will not cover a birthmark like this. Besides, such marks are usually considered interesting and are not covered. Other birthmarks, such as a strawberry mark or small broken veins, can be covered with the same cosmetic that was mentioned in the previous question.

PROBLEM: I have to wear glasses, and they make my eyes look as if they aren't there.

ANSWER: Plan to wear a little more mascara and eye shadow to play up your eyes under your glasses.

Makeup is fun to experiment with and fun to wear, and most young women will want to try it at some time or another. Just remember that you want to apply it so carefully that no one is really sure what or how much you are wearing.

3

TAKING CARE OF
YOUR SKIN

✎§ If you are old enough to be thinking about makeup, you are also old enough to start taking care of your skin. Glowing, healthy skin is a gift that will quickly fade if you do not give it proper care, and even troubled skin can be improved with proper care and attention.

For many years, the marketers of beauty products pitched their preparations to older women—those whose skin was already showing wrinkles and other signs of age. Today, cosmetics companies and doctors who specialize in skin care (they are called dermatologists) are more aware of the need for early and regular skin care. And please note the use of the word *regular*. It is useless to take care of your skin for one week, only to drop all pretense of caring for it the next.

How do you know when you are old enough to take regular, careful care of your skin? How do you know when the time has come to give your face a separate cleansing rather than the once-over in the shower that has been its usual treatment? Your body will usually tell you. About the time of puberty (nine to twelve years of age), your hormones become active in ways they have not been before. One result of this is a change in your skin. Its texture may change from the childlike softness to one slightly coarser. You may have occasional break-out problems—a blackhead or pimple may mar your complexion. This is when it's time to start a regular skin care program. Several are described in this book, and the one you choose should depend upon the condition and type of skin you have.

Understanding Your Skin

Before you can know how to handle your skin, you will find it helpful to know something about it. Basically, skin is composed of two layers: the epidermis, or outer layer, and the dermis, or inner layer. The epidermis is mostly composed of dead skin cells. In fact, it entirely renews itself every twenty-seven days. This layer of skin protects you from heat and cold, and it also takes the hard wear-and-tear that comes from both usual and abnormal use. Abnormal use, which we will discuss later in this chapter, refers to very hot and cold temperatures or pollution that may exist where you live. These unusual conditions all require some special skin care routines.

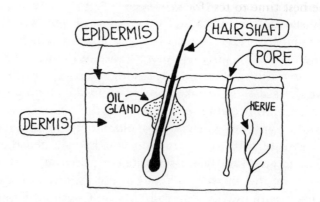

The dermis, or living section of your skin, contains nerve endings, small blood capillaries, glands that produce oil and sweat, and hair follicles.

One of the most important things to remember about your skin is that while you can apply creams and lotions to soften the epidermis or a mask to help slough off the dead skin cells, the things that matter to your dermis—and, therefore, to the health of your skin—are eating a good diet, drinking lots of water, and getting a lot of exercise.

What Type Skin Do You Have?

Because of the activity of the oil glands at puberty, most teens tend to have oily skin, at least for several years. As you age, your skin will probably become drier. Some teens, though, already have to battle dryness or a combination skin.

There are five skin types: normal, oily, dry, combination, and troubled. If you have troubled skin, you most likely know it already, for your skin has a tendency to break out with pimples and blackheads, and you may even have a fairly severe case of acne. The other skin types are easily discovered through a simple test and by observation.

The best time to test for skin type is first thing in the morning, assuming that you removed all makeup and cleaned your skin the night before. The only equipment you will need is some oil-blotting tissues, which can be purchased in any drugstore. Cut the tissue into four strips and apply a strip to your forehead, chin, one cheek, and your nose, pressing down lightly.

If you have normal skin, the tissues will stick and will not fly away. There will be no oily spots. Observation will show that you have barely noticeable pores.

If you have oily skin, the tissues will stick readily, and there will be oily patches on the paper. You have fairly large pores, especially around your chin and nose. Your skin frequently looks shiny, and you may have a tendency toward blackheads and other skin break-outs.

If you have dry skin, the paper won't stick at all. You will have small pores, and after washing your face with soap and water, it may feel tight. Your skin will also have a tendency to chap easily.

Combination skin is just what it sounds like—patches of oily skin mixed in with dry skin. If you have this type of skin, the oily areas will often be your nose and chin and possibly your forehead, and your cheeks will often be normal to dry.

Your skin color comes from the amount of pigment in your skin. Some people—black peoples, for example—have a lot of pigment. People with a lot of pigment tend to tan more easily than do fair-skinned people with little pigment.

Choosing the Skin Care Products that Are Right for You

So many skin care products are available that you would need a lifetime to try them all. Furthermore, many would not be suited to your skin. You have to find out which brands and products work best for you. Once you have purchased several skin care products, you have to devise a program for using them regularly. This will be discussed later in this chapter.

Here are the skin care products that you may want to use for your skin:

Cleansers. These can range from soap and water, to a special skin care soap, to a cream or lotion cleanser. If you have acne, your dermatologist may suggest special cleansers to use on your skin. Generally, dermatologists do not recommend using soap on skin that has started to dry out or that has dry tendencies. Most teenagers, however, have a slight tendency toward oily skin and can still use a mild soap and water.

Soap is a detergent, though, and because of its alkaline properties, it is believed to change the naturally acidic balance of the skin. Some doctors today feel that the skin's natural acidic balance is what helps prevent blemishes; other doctors pooh-pooh the whole idea and say soap is the only thing to use.

The wisest course of action, therefore, is to use soap if it feels good on your skin and doesn't aggravate blemishes or leave your skin feeling dry or raw. Avoid soap if it does not feel good to you. When washing, use lukewarm water and pat your face dry.

Cream cleansers usually have a lot of oil in them and are too strong for teenage skins.

Lotion cleansers are lighter and may be the perfect solution if your skin is slightly dry.

Under-makeup Lotions. While most very young teens do not need this, older teens may find that their skin feels better and takes makeup more easily if they smooth on an under-makeup lotion or cream first. Buy a very light lotion for this purpose

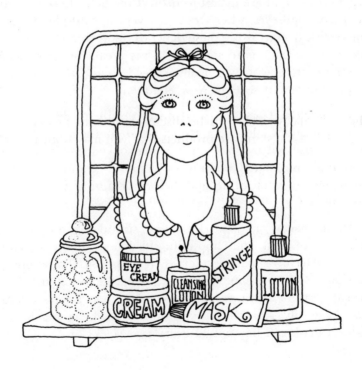

and use very little of it. Sometimes this lotion is enough to use for protection if you do not want to wear foundation, and it can also serve as an excellent, light night cream.

Night Creams. Most young women do not need to start using a night cream regularly much before their seventeenth or eighteenth birthdays, but you do need one then. Night creams come in two different formulas: oil-based and water-based. Water-based night creams are called moisturizers, because their function is to help keep the moisture in your skin. An oil-based night cream, too heavy for anyone under thirty or thirty-five, works to prevent and heal dryness. Moisturizers and night creams should always be applied to freshly cleaned, slightly damp skin.

Eye and Throat Creams. These are just heavier versions of night creams and are meant to protect the delicate skin areas of the throat and eyes, where there are very few oil glands. When you decide to start using these depends upon your skin type and age, but the trick is to start using any cream or lotion before you need it. Few young women need to use them regularly before the age of seventeen or eighteen.

Astringents. These are used on oily skin, to dry it slightly. Ask a cosmetics sales clerk to help you choose a gentle astringent, or use witch hazel on a water-soaked cotton pad or a combination of equal amounts of lemon juice and water. Apply astringent after cleaning and before creaming your face. Do not rinse off.

Masks. Facial masks work to tone, stimulate, and clean skin. The type of mask you choose should depend upon the type of skin you have; a makeup clerk will help you choose one that is right for your skin type. Grainy masks, often made from wheat germ or cornmeal, are especially good for oily skins. If you have oily skin, use a mask once a week; if you have dry skin, a mask can be applied every two weeks or so.

Taking Care of Your Skin

Every skin deserves a regular skin care program. First, it deserves a cleaning ritual. Cleanse your face at least twice a day, more often if you have problem skin. Second, it deserves protective treatment. Creams and lotions and masks are often applied at night, right after the final cleansing of your face. Creams and lotions are left on, while a mask is always removed after use. Read the directions on the package to see when to remove the mask you are using.

Finding the best routine for your skin, like finding the best products, requires experimentation. You may use soap and cleansing lotion in the morning and only lotion at night. Your skin may feel best with three thorough cleansings a day rather than two.

Remember, too, that a skin routine is not permanent. You should always stay alert to the possibility of changing a skin care program. Your skin changes all the time. As you get older, for example, your skin will get drier, and it will require extra creams. Your skin may break out around the time of your period, and you may want to take special precautions then. Skin exposed to summer sun and winter cold needs special treatment. Here are several standard programs for the various types of skin that can help you start planning your own individual skin care program.

Normal Skin Care Program

If you are blessed with normal skin, you don't have to do much with it during your teenage years except give it careful cleansing with soap and water or a mild lotion cleanser twice a day. Since normal skin is usually clear and pretty, you may want to skip foundation, wearing only a light lotion instead to protect your skin during the day.

Combination Skin Care Program

Treat this type of skin according to its separate needs. If your nose is oily, use an astringent on that area only. If your chin, cheeks and eye areas are dry, use a lotion or cream only on those areas. Usually combination skin needs a minimum of two good cleansings a day, using soap and water or a lotion cleanser.

Dry Skin Care Program

Although few teens have dry skin, most women eventually develop this type of skin. It is fragile and needs babying to look its best. Dry skin responds best to cleansing with lotion or cream. Soap and even water may only make the skin feel tight and uncomfortable. Dry skin always needs a protective lotion under foundation and a face cream at night. Eye and throat cream should also be used. Cleanse twice a day.

Oily Skin Care Program

Oily skin should be thoroughly cleaned as many times a day as it feels oily; usually this is three times. You can wash this type of skin in the morning, right after school, and before you go to bed. If your skin gets shiny during the day, you may want to carry small, premoistened towelettes to give it a quick pick-up. Soap and water are probably all you need for this type of teenage skin, although you may want to apply a light moisturizer around your eyes after the final cleansing of the day. Choose makeups especially developed for use with oily skins.

Troubled Skin Care Program

If you just have an occasional blackhead or pimple, you can handle this kind of skin without expert advice. If you have real blemishes that do not go away, you probably should see a dermatologist who specializes in treating teenage skin. Acne is no fun and has caused many young women a great deal of suffering.

Acne is caused by an increase in oil that is brought on by hormonal changes. Since the sexual hormones of the body become active at puberty, this is the time when most people have serious problems. Acne has no known cure. The best you can hope for is to control it and wait to outgrow it. Acne is not caused by food, although eating a balanced diet always helps keep your skin in top condition. Acne is not caused by dirt or pollution, but again, taking excellent care of your skin and cleansing it regularly will help to control acne.

Follow your doctor's advice if you are seeing one for your skin problems. If you are handling blemishes yourself, begin with two to three thorough cleansings a day. Do not use a detergent soap, but instead buy a soap especially designed for blemished skin. Use an astringent several times a week—once a day is probably too often. Avoid wearing makeup when you don't have to. Never pick at a pimple or blackhead—only a doctor or specialist in skin care is skilled enough to remove a blackhead or open a pimple without leaving a scar. A grainy mask, such as one made with cornmeal and milk or water, used once a week, may help a mild case of acne.

Above all, do not try your best friend's prescription lotions for her skin problems on your skin. Skin is easily damaged, and if you are going to use a prescription medicine on it, make sure it has been prescribed by your doctor for your skin.

Diet and Exercise and Your Skin

Your skin is only as healthy as you are—and healthy teens eat a balanced diet and get a lot of exercise. While no food is known to cause acne, your skin may have its own reactions to certain foods. Many skins break out from greasy foods such as potato chips or from chocolate. If you notice that a food tends to make your face break out, by all means avoid eating that food as much as possible.

31

Exercise is good for your skin tone and color. Try to leave time for serious exercise three or four times a week.

Climate and Pollution

Beauty experts are just beginning to realize what various climate extremes, sunlight, and the pollution in large cities can do to skin. For years, most women wanted to get as tanned as they possibly could during the summer—this was considered the ultimate in healthy looks. Now more and more people have come to realize that excessive amounts of sun, and even minor amounts of sun for those who are fair-skinned, are not healthy. Furthermore, sunlight has a cumulative effect on your skin. You may get tanned deeply four summers in a row, only to watch the tan fade over each winter. Still, permanent damage has been done to your skin, and it will take its toll in early wrinkling and a leathery look. If you care how your skin will look in twenty or thirty years, there is no better time to start taking precautions than during your teenage years. Take the sun in small doses, ten minutes at a time if you are fair, and thirty if you are dark. Wear a tanning lotion if your skin tans easily or a sun block if you have fair skin. Cream your skin carefully to moisturize it after any large doses of sunlight.

Skin may also need extra attention during the cold winter months. Wrap a scarf around your face before going out. Use extra creams and lotions to protect your skin before and after exposure to cold or windy weather.

If you live in a large city, pollution can damage your skin. Take extra care to cleanse your skin thoroughly. Under-makeup lotion and/or a foundation are musts to protect skin against city dirt, and a weekly mask is a necessity.

It's Never the Wrong Time to Start Caring for Your Skin

Ideally, a regular skin care program should be started as early as age ten or eleven. At this age, you will mostly want to form the habit of washing your face regularly. By sixteen or seventeen, you will probably be thinking about a special soap or lotion to cleanse your face, wearing a foundation to protect it during the day, and applying a light cream at night occasionally to combat dryness. By seventeen or eighteen, you should have developed a regular skin care program and should be protecting your skin against aging by using moisturizers and possibly eye creams. Remember, though, that you are never too young or too old to begin a regular skin care program. And remember that the beauty of your skin is more than skin deep—taking care of your general health does give you prettier skin.

4

A DAZZLING SMILE

~§ Your teen years are especially important for dental care because they (and, for that matter, your early twenties) are a time when you are especially prone to tooth decay. They are also a good time to form regular habits of dental care if you have not already done so.

Unfortunately, tooth decay and gum disease are not reversible. Unlike most diseases, they do not go away eventually with or without treatment, but rather, they become progressively worse as time goes on. Your best bet, then, for keeping your teeth pretty and healthy is a regular program of oral hygiene that includes visits to the dentist.

Why Teeth Decay

A discovery made only in the last few decades is that tooth decay is largely caused by plaque, a transparent film consisting of bacteria and saliva that eats away the enamel. Most teens only have to worry about decay, which is caused by one kind of plaque, but adults also need to worry about gum disease, caused by another type of plaque, which is the major cause of teeth loss.

Sugar—or any food containing sugar—also contributes to the formation of plaque, and if you care about your teeth, you will make a serious effort to cut down on the sugar in your diet.

While smoking is not a particularly major source of tooth trouble (however unhealthy it may be otherwise), it does leave your teeth stained and your breath smelling less than fresh. Over 27 percent of teenage girls smoke—which means you have a lot of years ahead of you in which to stain your teeth with tobacco. These ugly, hard-to-remove stains require extra visits to the dentist.

Visiting the Dentist

Dentistry today is quite painless. And you have even less reason to be frightened of a dentist if you know what to expect when you visit. Plan to visit a dentist every six months during your teen years, and more frequently if he suggests that you need it or if you have a toothache.

There are several ways to find a good dentist. Call the local dental association for recommendations, or call a dental school and ask if any of the professors have private practices. If money is a problem, consider going to the dental school; you will receive excellent care from student dentists who are supervised by teacher-dentists.

There are several ways to know that you have a good dentist:

• A dentist should discuss fees openly and be willing to let you pay off major work over a period of several months.
• He should explain what he is going to do to your mouth before he does it.
• He should talk with you about oral hygiene.

On the day of your appointment, you need only remember not to use mouthwash, as it disguises any problems you have with bad breath. Bad breath is a tip-off to the dentist of ill health or a need for dental care.

On your first visit, the dentist will probably take a brief medical history, ask if you have any allergies, and do a full set of X-rays. (If you are going to a dentist for the first time, you might want to ask him to get any recent X-rays from your old dentist.) X-rays, which should be rarely done, are necessary to show what is going on between your teeth and in the bone structure.

Basic Oral Hygiene

Brushing and flossing are the two major steps in dental care.

You should brush your teeth at least twice a day, more often if possible. Use a soft-bristled brush with rounded bristles, and a fluoride toothpaste. Pay special attention to the area where

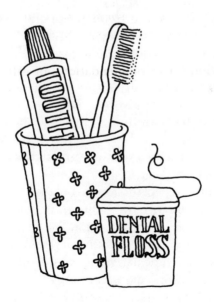

the teeth and gums meet when you brush. Brush with a small rounded motion, applying light pressure to your gums, and don't forget to brush the backs of teeth as well as the fronts. Reach for those out-of-the-way spots—they are exactly where decay is most likely to start. You can't do a good job with a worn-out toothbrush, so as soon as your brush looks the worse for wear, throw it away and buy a new one.

Flossing is a relatively new idea in dental care, but it goes a long way toward preventing the formation of plaque. Floss every night before you brush your teeth, then give your teeth their most thorough brushing of the day. There are numerous brands of floss on the market, and you may want to try several to find one that suits you. Buy unwaxed floss. To use it, take a 15- or 16-inch piece of floss and slip it in and out against the side of each tooth—including the hard-to-reach back teeth.

Special Dentistry

Most teens are aware of braces, since so many wear them. More correctly called orthodontia, braces refer to the correction of teeth through nonsurgical means. They are safe and relatively painless. Your regular dentist may suggest that you need braces, but they will be put on your teeth, if you do need them, by an orthodontist. Select an orthodontist with special care. Confer with him and get a second opinion before you make a final decision to wear braces. An orthodontist should have taken a two-year postgraduate course to prepare him for his work.

Basically, you need orthodontia because your teeth are not where they are supposed to be in your mouth—they are too crowded, too wide apart, or, most commonly, your bite is wrong. Orthodontia is not done for cosmetic reasons alone, but is a necessary if not urgent technique of rearranging your teeth so they can work more efficiently.

If you need braces, it is important to wear them while you are still growing, although in recent years orthodontia has been done with success on young adults. Orthodontia lasts from six or eight months to two years. It is expensive, costing anywhere from $1,500 to $3,000, depending upon the area of the country you live in. (If this is beyond your family budget, remember dental schools.)

Braces are metal or plastic wires that are fitted over your teeth. Sometimes they are wrapped around individual teeth, and sometimes they are stretched across teeth. The kind of orthodontia you need depends upon the type of straightening your teeth require. Sometimes rubber bands are used, too. Occasionally, one or more teeth are removed to make room for your shifting teeth before the braces are put on.

It is not true that your chances of decay increase while wearing braces, but braces do mean that you have to take extra care of your teeth. Here's how:

- Brush carefully after every meal.
- Consider using a water pick to flush out food that gets stuck in your braces.
- Don't eat chewy foods or hard breads; they may cause braces to break.

There are several other special techniques for tooth care. Capping is a way of artificially restoring a tooth that is chipped or of giving an unattractively shaped tooth a new look.

Plastic sealants are sometimes used on adolescents to help prevent tooth decay. They are painted on chewing surfaces only, which means you must still floss carefully to remove plaque between your teeth. They last for three to four years.

Fluoride trays are another device to help prevent decay in persons extremely prone to it. A special tray is fitted to the shape of your teeth. You fill it with a fluoride gel and wear it for several minutes a day to help protect your teeth against decay.

Scientists are working on a vaccine to prevent decay, but until it is ready for use on humans your best bet is to continue the oral hygiene and dental care practices just described.

5

TAKING CARE OF
YOUR HAIR

⚘ Every one of us wants a head of hair that is luxuriously thick and manageable—ready to be fashioned into the very latest hair style. Unfortunately, Mother Nature only rarely gives us this kind of hair. The windblown, full, curly style made popular by Farrah Fawcett-Majors in the mid-1970s is a perfect example of the kind of hair style most of us want—and few of us can have.

The kind of hair you have—curly or straight, thin or thick—depends upon the kind of hair your parents have. If your mother has curly, thick, coarse hair, and your hair is the same way, you know where you got the genes that determine the character of your hair.

What Hair Is

What you can do with your hair is determined by the kind you have. You may also find it helpful to know what hair actually is, so you can understand what is involved in keeping it shiny and healthy-looking.

Hair is 97 percent protein. Like your skin, it has a slightly acidic coating, which is believed to help keep it healthy and shiny. The hair follicle, which is buried in your scalp, is the living part of your hair. The hair that is growing on your head is actually dead. From this you should be able to understand how your diet and general health play an important role in the health of your hair. The hair follicle receives all its nourishment inside your scalp and determines how good your hair will look before it even appears on your head.

What Hurts Your Hair

Hair may be dead, but that does not mean it can be treated carelessly. Hair that is mistreated soon breaks or develops split ends. Some of the things that hurt your hair are:

• Too much brushing. Our grandmothers may have sworn by a hundred strokes a day to keep their locks shiny, but modern hair specialists say you should brush your hair only enough to style it and for a few minutes before you shampoo to loosen the dirt. Also, it's not a good idea to brush wet hair, as it tends to break easily.

• Pulling hair back into a ponytail. The barrette or coated rubber band (never use any other kind if you pull your hair back), plus the stress on the hair from being pulled back, will gradually damage your hair. This doesn't mean you can't wear your hair on top of your head in a ponytail. It just means you shouldn't wear it this way day after day for years.

• Too much heat. Even a lot of sunshine will dry your hair, as will hair blowers, curling wands, and electric rollers.

• Rollers you put in carelessly or rollers you sleep on. These can hurt your hair for about the same reasons a ponytail does.

Split ends are the first sign of damaged hair. Often the hairs break off around the top of your head, producing a halo effect. However angelic you may look, your hair is ill and needs instant attention. Split ends are caused by too much heat on the hair, teasing, and by strong permanent or coloring chemicals. You can help split ends by stopping whatever you do to your hair that is bad for it, and by regular conditioning.

Dandruff is another hair problem. A serious case of dandruff needs the attention of a dermatologist. Its symptoms are itching scalp and small white flakes that usually embarrass you by showing up on your shoulders whenever you are wearing dark clothing. A mild case of dandruff can be cured by using a special formula dandruff shampoo. Take extra care to brush your hair before you shampoo to loosen the flakes.

Not rinsing the shampoo out of your hair very thoroughly can cause mild flaking that looks like dandruff.

Taking Care of Your Hair

Regular hair care involves shampooing your hair just as often as it is dirty—every day if need be—and taking steps to correct damaged hair.

Select a shampoo that is suited to your hair type. If you have oily hair, you need a shampoo especially formulated to help it. Dry hair, which needs to be washed less often than does oily hair, requires a gentle shampoo. If you wash your hair every day, you might want to buy a gentle shampoo or dilute your regular shampoo with water.

How to Give Yourself a Professional Shampoo

Giving yourself a professional shampoo is easy. You need shampoo, a conditioner (whatever your type of hair needs), and a towel. The shower is perhaps the best place to shampoo your hair, but you can also do it at any available sink.

Start by brushing your hair for a few minutes to remove any loose dirt. (Then let your comb and brush soak in mild detergent while you shampoo.) Massage with your fingertips for a minute or two. Then begin the shampoo, following these steps:

1. Wet hair thoroughly.
2. Apply shampoo and work up a lather.
3. Leave shampoo on for about two minutes.
4. Rinse hair very thoroughly. Believe it or not, rinsing is the most important step in a shampoo. If you don't rinse your hair well, all the conditioning and styling in the world will not prevent it from looking dull and developing an oily coating within a day or two.
5. Apply conditioner according to the directions.
6. Rinse, rinse, rinse again, just as thoroughly as you did to remove the shampoo.
7. Towel-dry your hair to remove excess water before you begin to blow-dry or style it.

Conditioning Your Hair

You may think that hair conditioners are special treatments that you use on your hair once in a while. This is not true. A regular hair care program should include conditioning. This will help keep your hair manageable and can even change its texture so it is easier to style. Plan to make it part of every shampoo.

The type of conditioner you buy depends upon the kind of hair you have. Flyaway hair, for example, is helped by a creme rinse. Thin hair can be built up to look fuller with a conditioner that contains balsam and protein-builders. Oily hair needs a conditioner designed for use on oily hair—never use a balsam conditioner or a creme rinse on oily hair as it will only make it oilier.

Dry hair is the type of hair that most needs a conditioner and may even need penetrating deep-oil treatments every few weeks. Dry hair is usually damaged hair, so your first step is to find out why your hair is damaged and then stop whatever it is you are doing to cause the damage. Occasionally, though, someone just has dry hair naturally and is not doing anything to damage it. Nevertheless, dry hair and damaged hair should be treated the same way. Buy a shampoo and a conditioner designed for dry or damaged hair.

Dry hair also benefits from an occasional hot-oil treatment. You can buy a commercial deep-treatment product, or you can give yourself a homemade treatment. To give yourself a homemade treatment, you will need the following things:

⅔ cup of olive or other vegetable oil
pan in which to heat oil
plastic wrap
comb
bonnet-type hair dryer

Heat the oil gently—how much you use depends upon how long your hair is. Use a comb to part your hair into small sections and work the oil into each section close to the scalp and out to the hair ends. When finished, wrap your hair in plastic wrap. Sit under the hair dryer for thirty minutes. Wash your hair *very thoroughly* to remove all traces of the oil. Use your regular conditioner as the final touch.

Permanents, Straighteners, and Color

These are the Big Three—things you can do to your hair but should not do without giving serious thought to how they may affect the quality of your hair. All involve harsh chemicals. All are relatively permanent.

If you only want a body wave, if you have no coloring on your hair, and if it is in good condition, you can give yourself a home permanent. Get a friend to help you and follow the directions carefully.

If, however, you have coloring on your hair or you want a very frizzy or curly look, get a professional permanent.

Hair straightening is basically getting a permanent in reverse, but this process should always be done in a beauty salon.

The chemicals come into more direct contact with your scalp since no rollers are used, and they are left on longer than for a permanent, so professional assistance is necessary to avoid damaging your hair.

Hair coloring is another major change for your hair. Most teens today like the natural color of their hair and do nothing to it. If your hair is mousy colored, though, you may want to experiment with hair coloring. Although there are permanent hair colors that you can apply yourself, your best bet is to try a temporary coloring or rinse that will add shine and color highlights to your hair.

Styling Your Hair

Once you have gotten your hair in good shape, you can start thinking about its style. Your hair style should be a combination of what's fashionable, what looks great on you, and what your hair is willing to do. There's no use trying to go very curly if you have naturally straight hair. Why shouldn't you try to go with your natural look anyway, since that will be easiest for you and your hair? The days are long gone when you will select a hair style just because it's "in." If one style is very popular, and you really want to try it, have an honest talk with your hairdresser about how it will work for you. Then follow his or her advice.

Finding a Stylist

The first step to selecting a flattering hair style is to find a hair stylist that suits you and your hair. A friend's recommendation—if you like how the friend's hair looks—is a good way to find someone, or you can check out the salon in your community that seems to have a reputation for doing with-it hair styles for young people. Here are four ways to tell whether or not you have found a good hairdresser:

- Most good stylists will cut only wet hair.
- The hairdresser should cut carefully, sectioning your hair and taking as much time as is necessary.
- The hairdresser should listen to you and ask you about your lifestyle before the *two of you* choose a hair style.
- The hairdresser should show you pictures of hair styles, if you ask, and look at any pictures you bring in showing how you might want your hair done.

Once you have found someone to style your hair, try to develop a good relationship. Be willing to listen to what he or she says and suggests for your hair, but do not tell the stylist to do anything he or she wants to do to your hair—if you do, you deserve what you get.

A Style You Can Live With

Hair styles do change every year or so. Most young girls or teens, however, do not wear the radical new hair styles right away. And most teens are too busy to spend a lot of time maintaining a hair style. The best way to get a style you can handle is to avoid extremes and let your hair go its own natural way.

There are also some time-honored suggestions for ways to wear your hair to flatter your face shape, but today most popular haircuts can be adapted to any face shape. You will need to find the length of hair that suits you best. Incidentally, not everyone can grow hair that reaches halfway down her back. Your hair grows about 1/2 inch a month, and since hair is constantly falling out, you simply may not be able to grow your hair very long. If this is the case, take a cue from what you have to work with, and wear your hair short or medium-length rather than letting it look scraggly as it tries to grow out. Here are some more specific suggestions for ways to flatter your face shape and hair:

- If your face is long or you have a very pointed chin, your hair will probably look best at about chin-length or shorter.

47

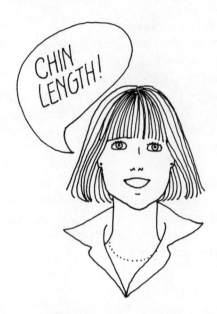

• If your face is square, try a soft, rounded effect to break up the square lines. Avoid straight-across bangs, flat hair on top, and an overly straight hairdo.

• If your face has round contours, you require narrow lines. Keep the crown fairly high and the sides close to the face. Slanted bangs help to break up the roundness.

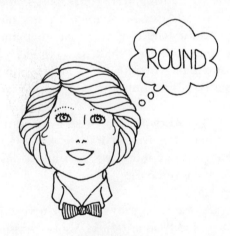

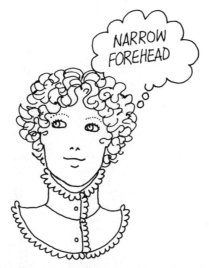

• If you have a narrow forehead, try fluffy width at your temples.

• Fine hair looks better medium-length; it is too limp and heavy to be worn very long.

• Curly hair quickly gets bushy if it is allowed to grow without styling, so always get a cut before you really need it.

• If you have a high forehead, bangs are your best bet.

• If you have a low forehead, avoid bangs.

• And by all means, if you have an especially pretty hairline, plan your hair style to show it off.

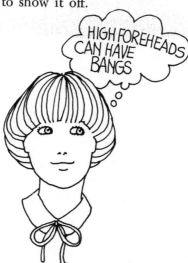

Hair Styling Appliances

Once you have gotten a new, flattering hair style, you will probably need to use one of three gadgets to maintain it: electric rollers, curling wand, or hair blower. There is a special technique to using each of these, and even this will vary depending upon the style you have chosen. When your hair stylist gives you a new look, watch carefully to see how he or she styles your hair so you can do it yourself later.

Here are some general hints on using electric rollers:

- The bigger the rollers, the looser the wave or curl.
- Do not leave the rollers in too long, or they will produce a ridge in your hair.
- Remove rollers slowly and carefully so you don't damage your hair.
- Let curls cool for a few minutes after the rollers are removed before you comb out—the set will last longer.

Here are some hints on using a curling wand:

- Your hair must be completely dry before you use it.
- Do not let the wand touch your scalp—it's hot and it could burn your skin.
- A too-hot wand will damage your hair, so be careful.
- Holding the wand in too long will also cause unattractive ridges in your hair.

Here are some hints on using a hair blower:

- Buy a professional model, if possible, one that uses 1000 to 1200 watts.
- Never use high speed to dry your hair—it will only damage it.
- Hold the blower at least six inches from your hair while using it.

• Keep the blower moving constantly while you style your hair.

• Leave hair just slightly damp rather than blow it totally dry—it's better for your hair.

In Conclusion

Taking care of your hair is a lot like taking care of your skin. You have to experiment to find what works best for you. And you have to be alert to needed changes in your hair care routine. Hair that is oily may go a little drier, and dry hair should always be given extra attention the minute it shows up. Watch the condition of your hair carefully and change your hair care routine as soon as you see any signs of change in your hair. Healthy hair should have lots of bounce and look shiny —when yours becomes dull and limp, start to think about taking better care of it or following a different hair care routine.

6

DAILY GROOMING—
MAKE IT A HABIT

◆§ If you are like most teenagers, you probably take a lot of teasing from your family over the length of time you spend in the bathroom getting ready to face your public. This may even be the cause of some friction. Yet, there is no doubt about it—looking pretty takes some extra time. Still, if you develop a regular beauty routine, there is no reason why you should spend more than twenty or thirty minutes a day on grooming. A daily grooming routine, after all, is a way of organizing your time. You still may spend some extra time in front of a mirror once you have worked out a routine, but you'll do it to admire the new you.

A daily routine will help you always to be well-groomed. You'll never have to turn down an invitation because your hair is dirty. Your nails will always look lovely, and your skin will always be pretty because of the constant care you give it.

A regular beauty routine consists of a few things you need to do every day in order to look your best, along with some special things that need to be done every week or a couple of times a month.

No one routine will work for everyone. If you have five

brothers waiting to use the bathroom, or you and your parents all have to leave the house at the same time every morning, this may not be the best time for you to set aside for your grooming. Maybe the solution is to take a little time after school for special things such as a manicure or pedicure, or to use the bathroom during the early evening.

Daily Grooming Habits

Here are a few things that you will want to do every day.

Bathing. Since you lead an active life, you will need a bath or shower every day and sometimes more often if you are actively involved in sports. Bathing can be the highlight of a busy day, for it gives you a few minutes to pamper yourself, relax, and think over the day's activities. A hot or cold shower will often give you the extra spurt of energy you need to get through a busy day or night.

Treat yourself to bubble bath if your skin is oily and to bath oil if you have a tendency toward dry skin. If you are planning to use a scent later, your bath oil should not be highly perfumed.

After the bath be sure to dry thoroughly in order to avoid chapped skin. This is the time to slather on body lotion or cream. Also use the towel to push back your cuticles gently. Doing this regularly will help you avoid hangnails.

Cleanliness is especially important during your period, when you may want to bathe or shower more often. You will probably feel better about yourself if you take extra precautions to stay fresh and pretty.

Deodorants and Antiperspirants. Another part of your daily grooming is using a deodorant. Many teens become upset and worried when they begin to sweat a lot. Both children and adults sweat—this is the body's way of regulating your temperature, among other things—but teenagers seem to suddenly become aware of it. Never fear—this is something you can easily handle. Buy a deodorant or antiperspirant and use it regularly. The product you buy depends upon how much you sweat. Deodorants protect against odor, and antiperspirants do this *and* also slow down the sweating process. Both deodorants and antiperspirants come in cream, lotion, and spray form.

Deodorant or antiperspirant should be applied right after your bath or shower. Cover your entire underarm with several coats.

Some vaginal spray deodorants are made for use during your period, when many girls worry about body odor. These are not particularly good to use. If you feel you need something extra during your period, buy some towelettes designed especially for this use.

Scents. At the same time that you apply body lotion and deodorants or antiperspirants, you may want to use a little of your favorite scent.

There are all sorts of ways that you can wear a favorite scent. The strongest scent you can buy is perfume; then comes toilet water; and finally, the weakest scent is cologne. Perfume lasts a long time, but it is expensive. Cologne, in fact, is probably ideal—it doesn't cost a lot and it isn't so heavy. Once you have chosen a favorite scent, you can usually buy matching bath powders and soaps if you like.

Apply cologne or toilet water to your wrists and neck. Be careful not to apply too much or it will quickly lose its charm.

To buy a scent, you simply must go to a store and try them on until you find one that suits you. Your nose wears out quickly, though, so you can only try on up to three scents at a time. Since every scent smells different on each woman, a good cologne truly does become your personal signature.

Hair—Getting Rid of What You Don't Want

It is interesting that European women do not shave their legs or underarms—to do so is considered unattractive. But in America women are generally considered attractive only if they do remove the hair on their legs and underarms.

When is the best time to start removing excess body hair? Whenever you feel uncomfortable with it. Body hair coarsens and darkens in color as you go through puberty. If you have light hair, you may notice less of a change and not feel particularly pressed to do anything. If you have dark hair, you may be worried about it and want to do something to remove it.

There are several ways to deal with unwanted hair—shaving, depilatory, waxing, electrolysis, and bleaching.

The best and easiest way to remove hair from your legs and underarms is by shaving. It's cheap, easy, and it involves no potentially dangerous chemicals. You simply use soap and lots of water. If you remove body hair by shaving, you will need to do this every day or every other day. Make it part of your bath ritual and you will hardly notice that you are doing it.

A depilatory is a chemical that melts the hair. You smooth it on, according to the package directions, and then remove it and the hair later. You only have to use a depilatory every two to three weeks.

Waxing, also a chemical preparation you can buy in a drugstore, involves melting wax and smoothing it on your legs, letting it dry, then pulling it—and your hairs—off. One waxing lasts six to eight weeks, but it hurts a little to pull that wax off. It works fairly well in small areas—for example, to remove excess hair from your face. Buy a waxing preparation especially suited for use on facial hair and use it according to directions. Always follow directions carefully when waxing, and it is even a good idea to ask your mother or a friend to help you the first few times you try it.

Another way to remove excess facial hair is through electrolysis. In electrolysis, an electric current is passed through a small needle inserted in each hair follicle. There is some discomfort, and the procedure is expensive as it can only be done by a trained professional. But electrolysis is something to think about if you have a lot of facial hair.

Perhaps the best and safest way for a teen to handle unwanted facial hair is by using a light bleach. After all, every human has facial hair, but the kind that causes the most worry is dark hair. You can buy the ingredients for a facial bleach from a pharmacist, or you can buy a commercial preparation. If you make your own, buy 20-volume hydrogen peroxide, ammonia water, and petroleum jelly. Mix 1 tablespoon 20-volume hydrogen peroxide with 3–4 drops of ammonia water and add enough petroleum jelly to make a paste. Smooth on your upper lip and leave on for about ten minutes. Wipe off and rinse the area with warm water. Apply facial bleach carefully, and take precautions not to get any in your eyes. Never use facial bleach on your eyebrows or eyelashes.

Care of Your Nails

Caring for your fingernails and toenails should be a regular part of your daily grooming routine. You will probably need a manicure once a week and a pedicure slightly less often.

The first time you paint your nails, you may not be successful. Practice is required to apply nail polish without any smears or smudges. Keep at it, though, and you will soon develop a steady hand. Here are ten steps to a perfect manicure:

1. Assemble all the equipment you will need:
   cotton
   small bowl of warm, sudsy water
   nail file or emery board
   orangewood stick
   nail brush
   polish remover
   polish, base coat, and top coat
   facial tissues
   hand cream or lotion
   cuticle scissors
2. Remove your old nail polish, using several wads of cotton and polish remover.
3. Using an emery board or nail file, shape your nails. If you use a nail file, do not use a metal one; rather, invest a

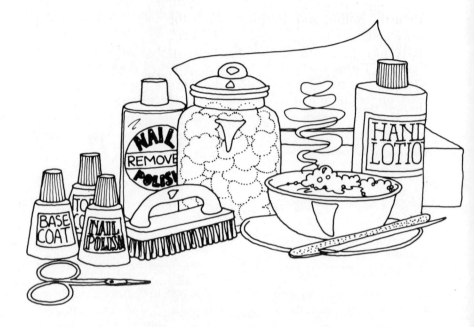

couple of dollars in a diamond file—it will last forever, and it
is even better than emery boards for filing your nails. File in
one direction only, especially if your nails are fragile, and work
for a smooth, oval shape. Overlong, clawlike nails require a lot
of care, and probably aren't worth the effort for any teen who
leads a busy life. They also scare boys, and may leave you open
for some teasing.

4. Use cuticle scissors to trim away any hangnails, if you
have them. Don't, however, use cuticle scissors to trim away
your cuticles.

5. Soak your hands in warm water for ten minutes.

6. Dry carefully.

7. Wrap a small piece of cotton around the orangewood
stick and gently push back your cuticles.

8. Rinse your hands at a sink and scrub gently with a brush
if necessary.

9. Apply polish if you want to, beginning with a base coat, then the polish, and finishing with a top coat. Consider using only clear polish except for special occasions—it is a particularly nice look. Teens look best in pale polishes—pinks and peaches—although you may occasionally want to experiment with brighter colors if they are in fashion. Very dark polishes look best on long nails.

10. Apply lots of hand lotion and massage into your hands for about five minutes. Manicure completed!

Foot Care

Few teens suffer from feet that hurt, and one way to make sure that you never do is to take good care of your feet, starting right now. Regular foot care should include a pedicure every week to ten days. Here are five steps to a perfect pedicure. Use the same basic materials you used for a manicure.

1. Remove old polish if you are wearing any, using cotton and polish remover.

2. Soak your feet in warm, sudsy water for ten minutes.

3. Cut toenails straight across, even with the tops of the toes, and then file to smooth out any rough edges.

4. Using an orangewood stick wrapped in cotton, gently push back the cuticles.

5. Apply new polish if you want to. To keep polish from smearing while it is drying, place cotton balls between your toes.

Always buy shoes that fit you and feel comfortable. A shoe should have one inch of extra space between your toe and the tip of the shoe.

You should also switch heel heights often, going from moderately high to flat heels or vice versa. It is hard on your foot muscles if you wear the same heel height each day.

Stop Biting Your Nails

Nail biting almost always becomes a source of embarrassment for a teenage girl. It is a hard habit to break, but you can do it if you try—and if you really want to. Here are five suggested ways to stop biting your nails:

1. Tell your best friend or friends you are going to stop biting your nails, and ask them to remind you each time they see you doing it.

2. Promise yourself a reward after you have stopped biting your nails for six weeks. Treat yourself to a professional manicure or buy some special accessory you have really been wanting.

3. Wear a loose rubber band around your wrist to remind yourself not to bite your nails. Give it a little snap instead whenever you feel the urge to bite your nails.

4. Give yourself a weekly manicure. If you go to all that effort, you may think twice before you undo it by biting.

5. Carry an emery board or nail file with you everywhere and use it any time you have a slightly rough edge on a nail.

Organizing Your Grooming Routine

Now that you know what you have to do regularly to always be well-groomed, you can spend a little time thinking about how you will fit these things into your life. Your teenage years are often very busy—school takes a lot of time, extracurricular activities become important, and you also begin an exciting social life. Most people who are successful socially and who accomplish what they want to in school learn very early to be organized—and setting up a grooming routine that works for you is one way of developing your organizational skills.

As mentioned earlier, you do need to take your family into consideration unless you have your own bathroom. A good grooming routine, however, should take no more than twenty to thirty minutes a day—and that includes putting on makeup. Here are lists of grooming rituals and how often they need to be done:

Daily
Bath or shower
Use deodorant or
  antiperspirant
Shave legs and underarms
Makeup
Exercise
Hair care

Weekly
Manicure
Facial mask (if your skin is
  oily)
Pedicure (during the
  summer)

Biweekly
Pedicure (during the
  winter)
Facial mask (if your skin is
  dry)
Deep conditioning or oil
  treatment for hair

Monthly to Every Six Weeks
Haircut or trim
Bleach or wax excess facial
  hair
General cleanup of your
  beauty supplies and
  drawers and purchasing
  of anything you may
  need for grooming
  routine

As you develop your own personal schedule, you will learn to fit in grooming routines with your other activities. You needn't do everything at once, but you will find you save a lot of time by having a regular routine.

7

SITTING AND STANDING PRETTY

⋖§ Anyone can move gracefully. It has nothing to do with how tall or short or how fat or thin you are. Moving gracefully is a learned motion—and with a little practice, anyone can learn how.

Sometimes, particularly with teens, awkwardness seems to hit suddenly. Occasionally it is imagined—you're suddenly thrown into a lot of new social situations or you may have just gotten your first real boyfriend, and your body seems uncomfortable with the whole idea. But sometimes the awkwardness is very real—as when you have just grown three inches in one year. Regardless of whether your awkwardness is real or imagined, it can be conquered, and you can soon be moving with an easy grace.

You should always walk, sit, and move to show yourself off. You need not be self-conscious about deliberately moving gracefully. At first it does seem strange to try walking or sitting a new way, but once you've followed our suggestions a few times your new way of moving will quickly become second nature. The advice that follows is designed to help you analyze how you move and to suggest the most effective and graceful ways of using your body. In addition to looking better, there is another reason to learn to move correctly: safety. While your body is built to do a lot of work and to use its natural strength, you can harm it by not moving correctly. People often try to move heavy things with their back muscles, for example, when they should really use the leg or arm muscles for heavy lifting and pushing.

Two Keys to Moving Gracefully

Although you will read specific hints on how to walk and how to do just about everything with your body, there are two general guidelines to follow no matter what you are doing. *First, keep your back straight.* Keep it straight while you walk, stand, sit, and do any other movement. Learn to lean forward from your hips when you reach for something; learn to lean forward from your hips when you are working at a desk— whatever you are doing, keep that back straight. *Second, keep flexible.* Good body movement does not involve rigidity. If you have ever had a chance to watch models at work on a runway, you undoubtedly noticed the ease and fluidity with which they moved. They are in good shape, their muscles are very flexible —and they are very graceful as a result. Flexibility also helps you to avoid being injured by overworking a muscle.

Taking a Good Look at Your Posture

Posture is how you place your body—not just when standing, but also when sitting, moving, and even lying down. Your posture reflects how you feel about yourself, and it also sends a clear message to the rest of the world. Teens who slump or shuffle their feet usually are telling the world they are unhappy or unsure of themselves. The teen who walks too quickly and rigidly is sending signals that she is too busy and unsure of herself to deal with other people. Quick, sudden movement also often shows aggression. Poor posture also may indicate that your feet hurt, that you need glasses, or simply that you are not well. Whatever the cause of poor posture, it is something you need to improve.

Before you can do anything to improve your posture, you must analyze what its flaws are. There are several ways to check your posture. Begin by putting on a leotard and standing in front of a full-length mirror. Observe where you bulge, whether your back is straight, if your tummy or rear sticks out too much. Ideally, you should ask a friend to take a photo of you standing exactly as you normally stand in profile. (Another method of analysis would be to go through old photographs and see if you are pleased with how you stand and sit.)

A less accurate method is to stand in profile in front of a mirror and imagine a string running down the center of your body. Does that imaginary string bisect your body? Does it run down the middle of your arm, hip, knee, and lower leg? If not, your posture needs improvement.

Here is another way to check your posture, or more specifically, your torso alignment: sit on the floor with your legs straight out in front of you. Have a friend place a yardstick along your spine. Your vertebrae should line up against it. If only the top of your spine touches it, or only the top and bottom touches, you have a posture problem.

There are other posture faults you need to check for.

Head. It should not protrude or be held too far back, with your chin tilting either up or down. In good posture your chin should be held parallel with the floor. Holding your head in another position puts undue strain on your neck.

Shoulders. Make sure they are not hunched, rounded, or pulled too far back.

Torso (upper body). It should not curve except gently between your neck and the top of your shoulder blades. Check for swayback or an accented arch in the middle of your back. Your spine should be straight between your shoulder blades and the end of the spine.

What to Do About Poor Posture

Sometimes poor posture is a result of not knowing any better. If this is true in your case, now that you know how you should stand, start practicing until good posture seems natural to you. Poor posture is also usually due in part to weak muscles of the back and neck. These can be strengthened through exercise. Here are some exercises designed to strengthen your back muscles.

Exercise 1. Lie on the floor with your arms stretched out overhead. Your knees will be bent slightly, so that the soles of your feet are flat on the floor. Pull in your stomach so the small of your back rests against the floor. Hold for a count of 10, then relax. Repeat 10 times.

Exercise 2. Lie on the floor with your knees bent and your arms bent at the elbow but flat on the floor at your sides. Straighten your arms and legs and, at the same time, pull in your stomach. Hold for a count of 10, then relax. Repeat 10 times.

Exercise 3. Here is an exercise to strengthen your neck muscles. Hold your head erect. Bend your face down slowly so your chin comes as close as possible to your chest. Bring your head to front position again. Slowly bend your head to the left. Return to starting position. Slowly move your head to the right. Return to starting position. Repeat 5 times.

Exercise 4. Begin with your head and jaw relaxed (yes, your mouth should be open). Drop your head to your chest and slowly rotate it in a circle 5 times. Return to starting position. Drop your head again and rotate 5 more times, this time going in the opposite direction. Repeat 5 times.

Almost any regular exercise will help you become more graceful, but walking and swimming are particularly helpful. Walking is good because you practice good posture while you walk; and swimming because you exercise almost every muscle of your body.

Working on Your Walk

After your posture, your walk is the most distinctive thing about how you move. In fact, your walk is like your signature —anyone who knows you wil be able to identify the sound of your walk before you come into view. The only question, then, is, what kind of signature do you have? Is it sloppy? Heavy? Shuffling? Too fast? However you walk now, you can easily improve with practice. The most time-honored exercise to improve a walk is to place a book on your head and walk around with it in that position for fifteen minutes. This worked for your grandmother and mother, and it will work for you.

Another secret to walking gracefully is to think tall. Pull yourself up to your full height, whatever it may be. Keep your shoulders loose and relaxed rather than artificially raised or hunched up. Pull in your stomach, and tuck in your rear end. Keep your legs comfortably flexed and relaxed rather than stiff.

Point your feet straight ahead rather than to either side, or to a slight outward angle if that is more comfortable for you. Keep your legs comfortably flexed and relaxed rather than stiff. down—not too hard—on the ball of your foot.

Whatever you do, don't shuffle your feet when you walk. Pick them up off the floor completely with every step.

The best way to get the kind of walk that will win you lots of admiration is to work at it. For several weeks, observe how people you admire walk, how models walk, and how actresses walk in movies and on television. Then go to work improving your own walk. It will seem a little strange at first—as if you are performing on stage, but soon your new walk will be totally a part of you.

Turning

Models are known for the slinky way they turn while modeling clothes. And while their motions are exaggerated and will mostly earn you laughs if you try to mimic them seriously, learning to turn—or pivot—correctly is a step toward gracious movement.

To pivot correctly, take several steps forward in a straight line, stopping with your right foot in front of your left foot. With your weight distributed equally on both feet, raise slightly onto the balls of your feet and make a 180-degree turn. Stop when your left foot, now in front of you, is straight and your right foot is at a 45-degree angle to your left foot.

Climbing Stairs

Among other things, climbing stairs is an excellent exercise for your thighs, and you should take every possible opportunity to walk up a flight of stairs. Shun elevators and escalators whenever possible. And when climbing stairs, do it right. Here's how:

- Keep your back straight.
- Keep your legs slightly flexed. Your large thigh muscles should be doing all the work here.
- Place your entire foot on the step. This keeps you balanced, utilizes thigh muscles, and avoids accidents.

Sitting

Always sit tall, though not rigidly. If possible, place the small of your back against the back of the chair in which you are sitting.

If you think about how you sit, you will probably find that you alter your posture, depending upon what you are wearing. If you don't already do this, it is something you might want to think about. You look better (thinner, more polite, if you will) sitting with your legs together. You can obviously sit with your legs somewhat apart or even cross-legged in jeans and pants, but do try to avoid looking like a lumberjack. Also, don't sit pigeon-toed. And once you have sat down, don't fidget. Easier said than done? You bet, especially if you're nervous about something or meeting someone for the first time. Here's a trick to appear relaxed even when you aren't: place your hands palm upward in your lap. If you are really nervous, grasp one thumb with the opposite hand or grasp a finger. You will still appear exceptionally calm and composed.

Almost everyone crosses her legs at one time or another. But if you must cross, try to do so at the ankles. Failing that, cross and uncross your legs fairly frequently, because sitting with your legs crossed for a long period of time cuts off your circulation. Also, don't risk crossing your legs while sitting on a platform or stage if you are wearing a skirt or dress. And remember that your legs look larger when crossed, so cross at your own risk.

Carrying Objects

No one looks poised carrying several objects, so the first trick—and it is one used by professional models—is to buy yourself a tote large enough to hold everything you have to carry—your notebooks, a couple of paperbacks, your sports gear, your makeup, everything. Then make sure that your arms do the heavy work while you carry—unless, of course, you have chosen to invest in a knapsack, in which case your shoulders will do the work.

Moving or Lifting Heavy Objects

Learning to lift heavy objects properly is a matter of safety as well as moving gracefully. Let your arms or legs do the work; pushing or lifting heavy objects with your back muscles only risks strain on them, so keep your back as straight up and down as possible.

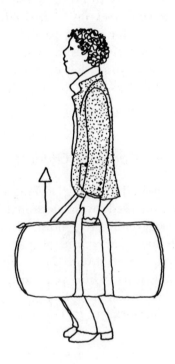

Getting In and Out of Cars

There ought to be an easy way to do this? There is: sit down on the seat with your feet outside on the ground, then swing them into the car, lifting them in front of you. Slide across the car seat, if necessary (try to avoid doing this—it's wear-and-tear on your clothes). Simply reverse everything to get out: place your feet on the ground, then lift your body out.

Putting a Coat On and Off

Almost as mysterious as getting in and out of a car is the art of putting on a coat and looking graceful at the same time. Yet there is also a technique for this:

1. Slip the coat slightly off your shoulders with a shrugging movement.
2. Reach behind your back and grasp one sleeve with the opposite hand (see illustration).
3. Slip off that side of the coat; the other side will follow naturally.

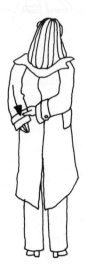

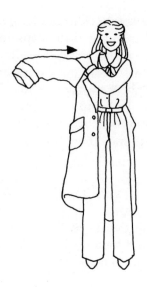

To put the coat back on:

1. Slip one arm into a sleeve.
2. Use the opposite hand (see illustration) to pull the coat over your shoulders.

Looking Graceful in Your First High Heels

Even if everyone knows that you are wearing your first pair of high heels, you still want to look like an old hand at it. The way to do so is practice. Wear the shoes for several hours at home before you venture out in public in them. They'll feel funny at first, but keep at it, and you will get the hang of wearing high heels. Simply remember everything you read earlier about posture and walking and follow the same rules when wearing your new shoes. Here are some other hints:

• Do practice until you walk just as you normally would.
• Let your arms swing naturally in directions opposite your feet; it will help your balance.

• Take steps somewhat larger than the length of your feet. Too many teens walk in mincing little steps in high heels— you need to practice regaining your normal walk. (If your normal walk *is* mincing little steps, you need to practice taking bigger steps.)

If, after several hours of practice, you still feel very off-balance, maybe these heels are too high for you. And if this is the case, you probably look silly in them, too. Retire these heels, and get yourself a pair of lower ones if at all possible.

Extra Help for Self-Consciousness

If after following the suggestions in this chapter, you still feel awkward, you may want to consider taking exercise or dance lessons several times a week. The regular exercise will stretch and develop your muscles, which, in turn, will give you added self-confidence. Taking up a new sport is another way to increase your self-confidence.

Protecting Your Eyes

While protecting your eyes may not seem to have much to do with how you move, most teens spend many hours reading and studying, and knowing how to sit properly when reading or working at a desk is important. When reading or writing, sit in a comfortable chair or, preferably, at a desk. Your back should be fairly straight or slightly curved. Your reading material should be held at about a 45-degree angle from you. Any other posture causes your eyes to distort to compensate for the angle, and it can cause permanent vision damage if you do it over a long period of time. You can see now why it is not a good idea to read in bed.

Your feet should comfortably touch the floor while you read or write. Avoid working at a surface much above or below your waist level. It is a strain on your back muscles and can also lead to vision problems.

Always read in a good light. Overhead lighting—the kind in most classrooms—is the best, but at home you should place a lamp slightly behind you and above your shoulder height. Avoid glare if possible and make sure the light does not cast any shadows. Good reading habits formed now will last a lifetime.

Practice Makes Perfect

Does this chapter seem like a long list of do's and don'ts? It really isn't, for once you have gotten the hang of moving right, it will become habitual and you will always move gracefully. And anyone can learn, with a little practice. Now is the time to begin.

8

EXERCISE FOR TEENS

⁂ An expert on obesity recently observed that overweight teens do not necessarily eat any more than their skinnier sisters. The big difference, he said, is that they get less exercise and are more sedentary. So if you have to knock off a few pounds and you are very sedentary, exercise may be the key. And even if you have no weight to lose, regular exercise is one of the best lifelong habits you can possibly develop.

Many teens get exercise naturally. You attend gym class, you play on a basketball team, you may love tennis and play it year round, or you may be a jogger. Whatever your form of exercise, you need to do it regularly. And if you do not get regular amounts of some strenuous exercise, then you need to think about creating an exercise program for yourself.

How Much Exercise Do You Need?

You probably cannot get too much exercise. Some teens just naturally get a lot of exercise; others get somewhat less but still play at some sport on a regular basis. If you do neither, and you're thinking about setting up your own personal exercise program, plan to allot two or three thirty-minute sessions of hard exercise per week. Ideally, even this should be supplemented by several hours of walking, bicycling, or some other routine sport.

The chart that follows shows how many calories you burn off doing various kinds of exercise. It should help you determine whether or not you are getting enough strenuous exercise on a regular basis.

Burning Off Calories with Exercise

Here is a list of activities teens are typically involved in and the amount of calories they burn off in an hour:

bicycling, medium fast	300
calisthenics	280
sitting in class	20
dancing	280
jogging	580
jumping rope, 80 skips per minute	500
running in place	450
roller skating	300
skiing, downhill	525
skiing, cross-country	620
yoga	200
swimming, crawl	250
tennis, singles	350
tennis, doubles	260
walking slowly	160
walking fast	325

How Much Exercise Is Too Much?

Can you overexercise? You certainly can, and a pulled muscle is not only no fun, but it takes several weeks—during which you should not use that muscle at all—for a torn muscle to heal. Your muscles should be stretched when you are exercising, but they should not actually hurt, nor should they become shaky. If either of these two reactions occurs, you are pushing yourself too hard and should relax and resume exercising at a slightly less strenuous level.

On the other hand, you should definitely feel a pull on your muscles when you exercise. If nothing is pulling, then you aren't working hard enough.

Will Exercise Alone Cause You to Lose Weight?

Probably not, unless you increase the amount of exercise you get by a very large amount. Exercise will decrease your appetite or at least help to keep it in balance. And you will look thinner because your muscles are tighter.

Developing a Personal Exercise Program

If you decide to develop your own exercise program at home, there are a few things you can do to make it more fun for yourself and to insure that you actually do form a habit of getting regular exercise.

• Buy a leotard or some other regular exercise outfit. Of course, you can exercise in underwear, but your routine will seem more serious if you have a special "outfit" to wear.
• Decide what equipment you need, then buy it. You won't need much. A blanket folded several times can serve as an exercise mat, or you may want to invest in the real thing (about $35–40). A jump rope is essential, as you will learn later. You may also want to buy some weights. Most teens work comfortably with 3- to 10-pound weights. Consider a set of barbells and some weights to put around your ankles and wrists. The extra resistance that weights provide makes any exercise you do that much more effective. All the exercises in

this chapter are done without the aid of weights, but any exercise in which you lift your arms and legs could be enhanced with weights.

• Except for the few exercise aids just mentioned, there is little else around that truly helps. Machines that bounce you around really do nothing in the way of stretching and toning your muscles. You will do better not to waste your time with these and to concentrate on serious, self-motivated exercises.

• If you plan to exercise at home, you will probably want some degree of privacy. Find a spot where you have enough space to stretch out comfortably and then plan to exercise when no one is around.

• On the other hand, exercising can be more fun when done with a partner or partners. Ask your mother or sister if she wants to join in your efforts. Having a family member join you is usually better insurance than a friend since your partner will always be nearby. Forming an exercise group with friends, however, is another means of motivation.

• Music often helps to set the mood when you are exercising. Play any kind that motivates you, although very slow or very fast music is probably not the best kind to exercise to.

• Change your routine fairly often. First, you should change it so you are always stretching your muscles more and more. Then, you should change your routine to prevent boredom. When you can do your exercises without giving them a thought, you are probably not doing them as thoroughly as you should—this is the time to reinvent your routine to give yourself a new challenge or more variety.

• Don't exercise right before you go to bed. It will only overexcite you and make sleep difficult.

• Develop a routine that exercises your entire body. You can do spot exercises to shape up your thighs, stomach, or your derriere if this is what you need, but the most benefit comes from exercise that works out the major muscles in your body. The exercise program that follows is designed to make you use all the major muscles of your body, and a few spot exercises are also provided for those special areas.

The exercises that follow consist of three sections. In the first section are the warm-up exercises that are necessary before you begin any serious form of exercise. These are very important, as it is not particularly healthy to work muscles that you have not prepared. Warm-up exercises consist of stretches and activities that start to loosen your muscles and make your heart beat faster than it usually does.

The second section contains a balanced set of exercises that can be used to develop all the major muscles in your body.

The third section consists of a set of exercises to tone up those hard-to-reduce parts of your body.

You can use any combination of these exercises to produce your own personal exercise program, or you may want to start by following the three-week diet and exercise program in Chapter 17.

I. Warm-Up Exercises

As you exercise regularly, you will lengthen the amount of time you are able to do these exercises. Ideally, you should do each one 2–3 minutes as part of the series of warm-up exercises.

1. Jumping Jacks. Do jumping jacks until you are tired, then do 5 more, and then rest 1 minute. To do: start with legs together, and as you jump lightly into the air, open your legs so you land with your feet about a foot apart; at the same time, bring your arms over your head and clap your hands together. Arms and legs should return to start position at same time.

2. Running in Place. Run in place until you are tired, then run 10 more steps (5 for each leg), and then rest for 1 minute.

3. Jump Rope. Jump until you are tired, then jump 5 more times, and then rest for 1 minute.

4. Body Stretches. Bend forward from your waist and stretch your arms out straight in front of you with your head between them. Reach with your arms. Straighten your back and pull

79

your back, arms and legs. Hold for 5 seconds. Relax. Repeat 5 times.

5. Arm Stretches. Hold your arms out perpendicular to your body. Move them in small circles for 1 minute. Reverse direction and repeat exercise for 1 minute.

6. Deep-Knee Bends. Placing feet a few inches apart and turned slightly outward, slowly lower yourself, lifting your heels off the floor, then lift yourself to start position again. Keep your back straight and your rear end tucked under. Repeat 10 times.

II. General Over-all Exercises

These exercises increase flexibility and large muscle strength.

1. Toe Touches. Stand with arms overhead and feet comfortably apart. Keeping your legs straight, stretch one arm up and over and down to touch the opposite toe. If you cannot reach your toe, repeat exercise, stretching as far as you can, until you eventually do touch your toes. Reverse exercise, using other arm. Begin with 3; work up to 20.

2. Lunges. Stand with feet comfortably apart and arms held, as shown, at sides but out from body. Bend right knee, shifting

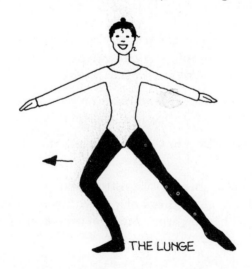

THE LUNGE

weight to that leg as you bend and keeping your left leg straight. Switch to left leg and repeat. This exercise is done slowly, and you feel a pull in your thigh muscles. Begin with 4 lunges (2 on each side) and work up to 10 on each side.

3. Sit-Ups. Lie flat on back with arms stretched out over your head and above it. (Alternate positions that will increase benefit of exercise include clasping hands in back of your head and crossing your arms over each other to grab opposite shoulders.) Breathe deeply, and as you exhale, lift yourself up slowly to a sitting position. Straighten your arms in front of you, or keep them in one of the alternate positions. Slowly return to start position. Begin with 5, work up to 15.

4. Thigh Stretches. Sit in position shown, with back straight and one leg stretched behind you. Place hand on leg that is stretched back. Slowly lean back as far as you can. Return to start position. Repeat 4 times for each leg; work up to 10 times. Note: Do not do this exercise if you have any knee problems.

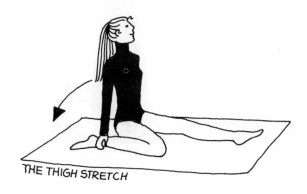

THE THIGH STRETCH

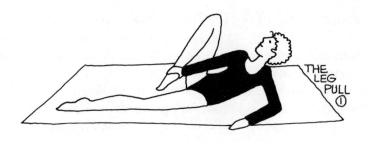

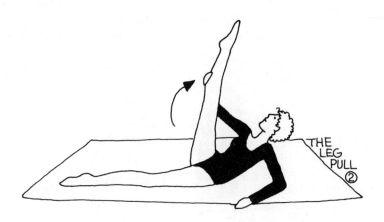

5. *Leg Pulls.* Lie on floor in position shown. Bend one knee
and hold foot with hand; your arm should be straight. Slowly
lift your leg, sliding your arm down to your calf as you do so.
Hold for count of 5. Return to flexed-knee position. Repeat 5
times and work up to 10 times. Reverse and do with opposite
leg.

6. Leg Stretches. Start with both knees on floor, with body supported by knees and arms. Keep your back straight and your head up. Push your right leg out behind you, and then swing it down so your knee touches your chest. Repeat 5 times with right leg and then repeat exercise with left leg. Work up to 10 times for each leg.

7. Leg Raises. Lie on your back with arms stretched out perpendicular from your body. Bend both legs at knees in start position. Slide one leg down to the floor and then slowly lift it as high as you can, keeping leg straight but not rigid. Return leg to floor, also slowly, and then to bent-knee position. Do exercise with other leg. Start with 4 times on each leg; work up to 10 times. Note: Do not raise both legs at the same time as this could hurt your back.

8. Side Stretches. Stand with your feet slightly apart. Place your left arm at your side touching your thigh and your right

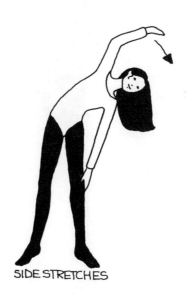

SIDE STRETCHES

arm over your head, as shown. Bend to the left until you feel a pull in right side. Bounce gently a few times. Release. Repeat 5 times and work up to 15 times. Repeat exercise on other side same number of times.

9. Push-Ups. Lie on your stomach with your palms flat on the floor, just below your shoulders. Using your arms and shoulders, lift your body off the floor, keeping your back and legs straight. Slowly lower yourself in this position, but do not rest your body on the floor. Begin with 2, work up to 10.

10. Balancer. Stand with your back straight, and feet together. Pull your left leg sideways, with your knee out, your foot resting against your thigh, and your left hand holding your ankle. When you have reached this position, hold, inhale deeply, and

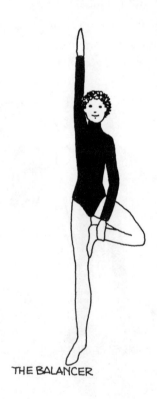

THE BALANCER

stretch your right arm straight above your head. (See illustration.) As you exhale, bend over, leaving your left knee bent, and touch the floor with both hands. Reverse exercise, using bent right knee. Work up to 3 times each side.

III. Spot Exercises

1. Stomach Pull. Lie flat on your back, arms at your sides. Inhale and lift your legs slowly about 1 foot off the floor. Hold for count of 5. Return slowly to start position, exhaling as you do. Start with 5 and work up to 20.

2. Hips, Thighs, and Derriere. Lie on floor in start position, with one arm over your head and the other supporting your body. Lift left leg slowly and then return to start position. Repeat 5 times on one side and work up to 15 times. Repeat exercise on other side.

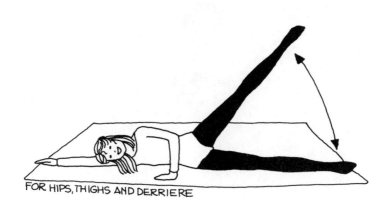

FOR HIPS, THIGHS AND DERRIERE

3. Waist Reducer. You need a fairly heavy book or a 5-pound weight as equipment for this exercise. Stand straight with feet slightly apart, and hold a book at one sid . Bend gently, letting book pull you down, and bounce several times. Return to start position. Place book in other hand, and repeat exercise on that side. Start with 20 bends on each side and work up to 40.

4. Chest and Shoulders. This isometric exercise involves applying pressure by squeezing your hands together, which causes a pull in your arms and back. Push arms together, as in the illustration. Then, push arms together and, at the same time, push them upward, although you should *not* actually *move* your arms upward. Repeat each exercise 10 times and work up to 25 times.

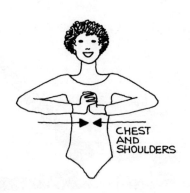

CHEST
AND
SHOULDERS

5. *Hip and Thigh Muscles.* Lie on the floor as shown. Support your upper body with your arms. Raise your leg, as shown, and bend it from the knee 10 times. Reverse sides and repeat exercise. Work up to 20 times on each side.

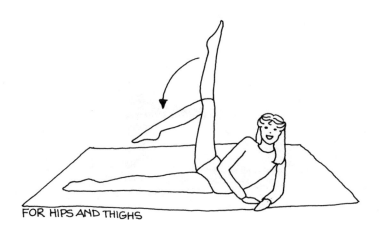

FOR HIPS AND THIGHS

6. *Thigh and Stomach.* Lie on your back, arms perpendicular to your body. Swing one leg up, keeping it straight but not rigid, and then swing it down to opposite side. Try to touch fingers on opposite side. Keep your shoulders flat on the floor during exercise. Switch legs and repeat exercise. Do 10 times on each side and work up to 20 times.

7. Derriere. This exercise does not feel like work, but it does the job. Sit on floor, as shown, with arms stretched out in front of you. Your legs should be straight out in front of you. In this position, slowly "walk" forward on your rear end. Take 20 "steps" forward and then move backward.

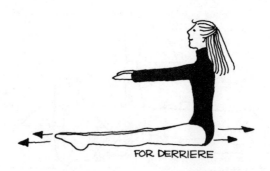

FOR DERRIERE

8. Legs. Lie flat on your back with arms at your sides. Press your hands to the floor as you do the exercise. Lift your legs and bicycle quickly, staying in place. As an alternate, you can lift your hips and support them with your hands, keeping your elbows flat on the floor. Start with 20 rotations and work up to 40.

9

NUTRITION

⋙ Your mother or a home economics teacher has probably told you—perhaps too many times—that you are what you eat. So why mention it again? Because it is absolutely true. You reflect what you put in your mouth in many ways. When you eat a healthy, balanced diet, your skin is clearer, smoother, and moister. Your hair has more shine and bounce. Your body tone is better, you feel better, and you have more energy. And learning to eat properly only requires that you know a little about nutrition.

Nutrition begins at the moment you are conceived. An embryo draws its nutritional needs from its mother's body, which is the reason that pregnant women are encouraged to eat well-balanced diets. From the moment you are born, what you eat also influences how you look and feel—as most parents are well aware.

Because small children usually eat as much as their parents allow them to eat, doctors have only recently become aware of the connection between fat parents and fat children. This is not a return to the outdated notion that fat is inherited—it almost never is!—but, rather, is a recognition of the fact that small children quickly take on their parents' eating habits. That's why fat parents often raise fat children.

By the time you are a teenager you are beginning to have some control over what you eat. You are also still flexible enough to change your eating habits totally if you want to. And if you weigh a little too much because everyone in your family does, now is as good a time as any to shed those extra pounds. Chapter 10 contains special diets for teens who need to lose or gain weight, along with hints on dieting. In this chapter, you can learn the basic information about nutrition that will help you always to be a wise eater.

Today's teens are more fitness- and health-conscious than those in any preceding generation. More information about our bodies' nutritional needs is available than ever before, so there is little reason for you not to know and do what is right for you nutritionally.

Nutrition is the study of the foods your body needs to maintain itself. Not too long ago, many people suffered from nutritional diseases because no one was quite sure what foods the human body needed. Even with all the advances that have been made today, food experts are not completely sure what the body needs. They do know this: you need some food every day in regular servings, and what you eat should provide you with a certain amount of protein, carbohydrate, fat, minerals, and vitamins. Many minerals and vitamins are only required in minute amounts, but they are still important and necessary, and others are needed in larger, regular amounts. There are probably some other food elements needed by the body that have not yet been discovered in laboratory testing.

How Much You Can Eat

Then, too, each person has her own rate of metabolism—this is the intricate process by which your body maintains itself. Most people's metabolisms fall into the normal range, but some have unusually slow or fast metabolisms. Even within the normal range, each person's metabolism is unique. For example, your best friend, who is six inches taller than you, may be able to eat a lot more food than you can without gaining weight. Another friend, who is nervous, may be skinny no matter what she puts in her mouth. She probably burns a lot of extra calories just being nervous. Then, too, small persons normally burn fewer calories than large persons do. What this means is that you must decide how much food you personally require to be well-nourished. Your metabolic rate may even change from year to year. If you have a sudden growth spurt when you are fourteen, you may find that you need more food than you did a year earlier when you grew less. By the time you are sixteen, if you have pretty much stopped any rapid growing, you may need a little less food.

Calories—How Many You Need

The energy that food supplies to our bodies is measured in calories. In order to lose one pound of fat, our bodies must burn up about 3,500 calories. Occasionally a diet is set up based on some other measure—fat portions, or servings of carbohydrates, or whatever. The safest and most time-honored way of measuring what goes into your mouth, however, is to count calories.

The caloric needs of a teenager are pretty set, and if you are dieting to lose or gain weight, you should not vary greatly from these amounts. Teens under sixteen should not eat fewer than 2,000 calories per day, and teens over sixteen need at least 1,700 calories per day. Many teens need closer to 2,500 calories a day from a balanced diet in order to meet their energy needs.

Eating a Balanced Diet

The notion of what a balanced diet is has shifted somewhat over the last fifty years, as medical research uncovered more about our needs. Basically, though, a balanced diet consists of meeting but not exceeding your caloric needs, eating a wide variety of foods to insure that you get all the nutrients you need, and eating these foods on a fairly regular basis—usually in three meals a day.

Americans and the Foods They Eat

Let's talk sensibly for a minute about the foods you need to eat to be healthy—it's an important issue in America. Americans are confronted with one of the world's largest assortment of junk foods and prepackaged foods, some of which are good for you and some of which are not. Americans are also obsessed with dieting and tend to attach themselves to any fad diet that comes along, whether or not it supplies their daily food needs.

You need to adapt a strategy for healthy eating in the midst of all this. Why is this so important for teens? Because your food needs are not the same as those of an adult. In addition to gaining or losing weight, you must cope with the fact that you have probably not completed your growth yet, and so you have special nutritional needs that must be met.

Fortunately, it is not all that difficult to meet your nutritional needs *once you understand what they are.* If you eat wisely—and this means eating a variety of servings from the basic food groups—you are probably well-nourished. Eating a balanced diet is nothing to be overly obsessed about. If you eat a little less bread than you should for a few days, you will not suddenly become malnourished. If you develop a craving for fruit one week and have five servings a day instead of four, you will not throw off your body's nutritional balance. A good way to insure getting a balanced diet is to become familiar with the basic food groups and the amounts recommended for daily consumption.

Basic Food Groups

Servings Per Day	Food Group	Kinds of Foods to Eat
4 (8 ounces each)	dairy	milk, cottage cheese, cheese (Note: 1 ounce cheese equals one serving.)
2 (4–7 ounces each)	protein	meat, fish, poultry, eggs, dried peas and beans, nuts (Note: 2 eggs equals 3 ounces meat, as does ½ cup dried beans and 1 ounce nuts.)
3 (about ¾ to 1 cup each)	vegetables	green beans, broccoli, spinach, lettuce and other salad greens, zucchini and other squash, tomatoes, potatoes (Note: One serving must be a leafy green vegetable; one, a yellow vegetable; one, a potato.)
2 (pieces, at least one high in vitamin C)	fruit	apples, oranges, pears, grapefruit, melon, peaches, tomato*
4 (¾ cup or 1 slice bread)	grains	bread, rice, oats, wheat, cereal

* Tomatoes, technically a fruit, can count as either a vegetable or a fruit in a balanced diet.

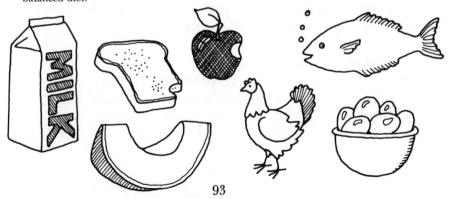

93

Vitamin and Mineral Needs

Your body also needs regular amounts of vitamins and minerals. Both are normally obtained by eating a balanced diet, although you may want to supplement your diet with a one-a-day vitamin pill plus iron. Some people take vitamins and minerals in individual portions, but this is a very complicated business, particularly for a growing teen, and, unless advised to do so by your doctor, it is better not to supplement your vitamin and mineral needs in this way during your teen years.

Food Myths—What They Really Mean

Americans have many—and sometimes strange—beliefs about food. Some of the myths are related to diets; others are about foods that are thought to be "good" or "bad" for you. Here are some of the more common food myths and the true facts about them.

Myth: All junk foods are bad for you.
Fact: Some junk food is healthy.
The hamburgers sold in fast-food restaurants do have some nutritional value, although you can't live on a diet of hamburgers only and expect to be healthy. The really bad junk foods—the ones with little or no nutritional value—are such things as candy, which consists largely of sugar, and potato chips and pretzels, which are high in salt and are also so filling that they may keep you from eating good foods.

Myth: Chocolate makes acne worse.
Fact: No one food has been proven to make acne worse.
You may find that a certain food tends to make your skin break out more often, and you should, of course, avoid any such foods once you have discovered what they are. But there

is no food that is known to make *all* cases of acne worse in *all* people. If you have problem skin, you just need to be extra careful to eat a balanced diet.

Myth: Margarine is healthier than butter because it contains fewer calories.
Fact: Margarine and butter each have the same amount of calories—about 100 per tablespoon.

Myth: Grapefruit helps burn off fat and is a special "diet" food because of this.
Fact: Grapefruit is just like any other fruit—a good source of vitamin C—and it has no special powers to burn off fat.

There are no magical diet foods. As we will discuss in greater detail in the chapter on dieting, the best way to take off pounds or to gain weight is through reducing or increasing the amount of food you eat.

Myth: Yogurt, honey, and brown rice, among other foods, are special diet foods that will help you lose weight or become a healthier person.
Fact: These foods are suitable as part of a balanced diet, but they do not have enough food value by themselves to provide a balanced diet.

Eating a diet of one of these foods exclusively could be injurious to your health.

Myth: Starch, found in breads and potatoes and rice, is bad for you.
Fact: Starchy foods are a good source of energy and are a necessary part of a balanced diet. They are better for you than foods with lots of sugar.

These, then, are some of the basic food myths that you are likely to hear. As new "fad" diets develop, you will undoubtedly be introduced to new fad myths. Your best defense against falling for a fad diet or food—something that might in the long run hurt your health and looks—is to always try to eat a balanced diet and a variety of foods.

In chapters 8 and 10, the roles of dieting and exercise in weight control are discussed in greater detail. Understanding some of the basic facts about nutrition should help you choose a diet that is suited to your metabolism and your lifestyle.

10

DIETING FOR TEENS

◄§ Almost no one thinks her shape is just right, that she could not benefit by losing or gaining a few pounds. Yet we all come in an amazing variety of shapes and sizes. The teen who looks pudgy at age thirteen may turn out to have very attractive curves at sixteen. The person who thinks she is just too skinny for words may find all those angles softening into curves during the course of a few months. Sometimes, though, you *are* carrying too many pounds around—or you may need to gain a little weight.

How to Tell If You're Too Thin

Many teens who just haven't filled out yet think they are too thin, so before you decide to make a conscious effort to gain weight, get an expert opinion. Ask a good friend, your mother, or better yet, a family doctor, if you should consider putting on some weight. Check the weight and height chart in this chapter. If your body weight is 10 percent or more below the recommended weight shown on the chart, you might want to consider deliberately adding a few pounds.

Weight Chart

This chart shows normal weight range for corresponding heights. You should weigh yourself unclothed. If you are small-boned, you will probably weigh on the low side; if you are large-boned, that is a reason for you to weigh in at the high side of this chart.

		Pounds	
Height	**Low**		**High**
4'7"	73		81
4'8"	87		95
4'9"	88		96
4'10"	90		98
4'11"	92		100
5'	96		104
5'1"	97		105
5'2"	100		108
5'3"	104		112
5'4"	108		116
5'5"	111		119
5'6"	116		124
5'7"	120		128
5'8"	125		133
5'9"	130		138
5'10"	135		145
5'11"	140		150
6'	145		155

You should also consider whether or not you have begun to develop an adult body. Many teens find that they suddenly have trouble keeping weight off once their hormones activate at puberty. If you are twelve or thirteen and a late bloomer, wait another couple of years. At sixteen or seventeen you are closer to being through puberty, and if you still feel you are skinny, then try to put on some weight.

How to Tell If You're Too Fat

The best way to tell if you weigh too much for your height is to consult the chart in this chapter. If your body weight is 10 percent above the recommended weight for your height, you may need to take off some weight. Also, strip down and look at yourself critically in a full-length mirror. If you see too many bulges where your body should be smooth, that's another sign. Pinch a piece of skin around your midriff—if you can gather up more than one inch of extra fat, you probably need to lose some weight.

Mothers and family doctors often tend to think of those few extra pounds carried during the teen years as baby fat—something that everyone hopes will eventually melt off of its own accord. This may happen, and then again, it may not, so if you feel burdened by your extra pounds, by all means now is the time to shed them.

If you weigh 20 percent or more than your suggested weight, you have a more serious diet problem, and you should see a family doctor or a doctor who specializes in dieting and plan a healthy diet with him. If your family doctor seems uninterested in helping you diet, ask him if he can recommend a nutritionist who will work with you to take off the weight. You could also try joining Weight Watchers or some other group designed to help people lose weight.

Analyzing Your Eating Habits

The best way to begin a diet is to analyze why you eat so much, as well as when and how. There are several reasons for weighing too much. The most common ones are:

- Your family eats a lot of heavy, starch-laden meals.
- You always have desserts or some kind of sweets during the day.

99

• You are addicted to soft drinks and drink at least one every day, sometimes more.

• You snack, possibly even eat an extra meal, after school and between dinner and bedtime.

Do you overeat for one of these reasons? Or for another reason? Keep a written record of everything you eat and the time you eat it for two weeks. Note the foods that are eaten during regular meals and the foods that are purely between-meal snacks. During this two-week period, eat as you normally would, or it won't be a fair record of your eating habits. Keep another record of the time you spend in heavy physical activity.

Why Diets Are Necessary

Most of us need a planned diet in order to lose weight. You may only need to lose a few pounds, which technically means you need only cut out a small amount of food, but few of us have the innate willpower to simply push ourselves away from the table on a regular basis. A diet is a means of providing the structure that keeps us from eating. And for teens, a diet is a way of restructuring eating habits at an age when you are flexible enough to maintain those habits for the rest of your life. Dieting is a lifetime process—once you have lost extra weight, you can go off the "official diet," but you should always be on a common-sense diet. And you should always be prepared to cut back for a few days the minute your weight starts to creep up again. Diets are hard work, and it's a shame to put yourself to all that work and fail to maintain the benefits.

If you get under five hours of exercise a week and you consume much more than 3,000 calories a day on a regular basis, either or both of these situations may be why you are overweight. And you are probably a good candidate for a diet.

Special Energy—and Diet—Needs of Teens

Teenagers are not yet adults physically. While an adult needs the energy provided by food to get through his or her regular round of daily activities, you use food to meet your energy needs *and* to grow. And growing, as you well know, is a very important activity. For this reason, you would do well to avoid any kind of fad diet. Most fad diets—which emphasize too much of one food or recommend consuming liquids only, for example—are not particularly good for most adults, and they are never a good idea for a growing teen.

There is another very good reason to avoid fad diets. You may experience a sudden weight loss through one of these diets, but you have not *changed your eating habits.* This means that the minute you go off a fad diet, or within a short time, you will most likely resume your poor eating habits and begin to regain the lost weight. Experts in weight control admit that they are not sure why people overeat, but more and more they are beginning to realize that the most effective methods of dieting are those that involve retraining one's eating habits. And it is certainly easier to retrain your eating habits when you are thirteen or fifteen than when you are thirty or forty.

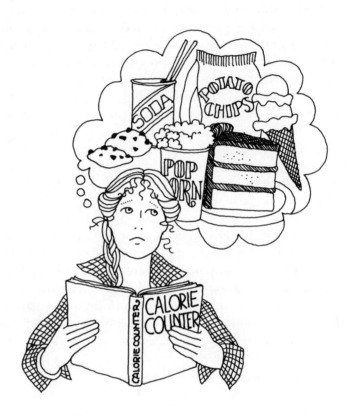

Counting Calories

The single most effective and time-tested way to lose weight is to reduce your caloric intake—to count calories, in other words. A calorie is a unit of measure, like an inch or a pound. It measures the amount of energy in a food and the amount of energy you burn up. One pound of fat equals 3,500 calories. That means you have to reduce your caloric intake of food by 3,500 calories to burn off one pound of body fat.

Sensible Lifetime Dieting

The diet on the following pages is really a way of eating. You do count calories, but rather than having every single food for each meal outlined in detail, you choose from lists of food groups. When you have reached the number of calories you need per day, you stop eating.

Most teens eat and exercise enough to handle 2,500 to 3,000 calories a day. If you weigh too much, you need to cut back from this amount. Teens over sixteen can safely cut back to 1,700 calories per day; teens under sixteen can cut back to 2,000 calories.

You can also use this diet plan if you want to gain weight. The trick is to increase the number of calories you consume. It is possible to gain weight by eating anything you want— ice cream, hamburgers, and lots of pretzels and potato chips. A *better* way, however, is to increase your caloric intake of healthy, nutritious food. Keep a record of the amount of calories you consume and then plan to add systematically to that number by eating extra food from the Food Lists that follow. For example, if you really like fruit, add a couple of extra servings of that to your meals. Add extra milk or even a milk shake before you go to bed. Within a few weeks, you should be gaining some extra weight.

The Food Lists in the diet plan are nothing more than foods (and their caloric values) taken from the Basic Food Groups Chart described in Chapter 9. Plan to eat the number of servings required on the chart (see page 93). Each day, or each week if you like, draw up menus based on these Food Lists. If you are cutting your caloric intake to 2,000 calories, select enough food to add up to 2,000 calories. If you are cutting your intake to 1,700 calories, plan to stop eating when you have reached that amount.

You have to do a little extra planning on this diet, but being involved with what you eat will make it easier to stay on the diet. This diet also permits you to eat a wider variety of foods than you would on an organized diet. It also means that you can eat what your mother cooks rather than demand special foods to meet your diet. (Of course, if your mother cooks a lot of pasta or other fattening foods, you might want to talk to her about this and enlist her aid in preparing foods that are lower in calories.)

If you do want to follow a more stringent diet for a while (sometimes this extra discipline helps), turn to Chapter 17 and follow the three-week diet and exercise make-over program.

How Fast Will You Lose?

When dieting, keep a record of your weight loss. But don't make the mistake of weighing yourself every day. Weight simply does not drop off that fast. At most, you can expect to lose 1½ to 2 pounds a week, and there will be times when you will reach plateaus and won't lose any weight for that week. When you begin dieting, you may also drop 5 or 6 pounds in one week. It's a nice bonus, but most of the lost weight is water, not fat. Enjoy it, but don't count on losing that much every week.

Weigh yourself once a week and record your weight on a chart that shows your progress.

Food Lists

Fruits

apple, raw, medium	75
apricot, raw	25
apricots, dried, 3	40
banana, medium	100
blackberries, ½ cup	60
blueberries, ½ cup	55
cantaloupe, ½ melon	60
cherries, raw, 1 cup	80
grapes, green seedless, 1 cup	105
honeydew melon, ¼ melon	35

nectarine, raw	60
orange	70
peach	40
pear	100
pineapple, raw, ½ cup	35
plum	20
prunes, dried, 4	70
raisins, 1½-ounce box	100
raspberries, ½ cup	30
strawberries, 10 large	35
strawberries, 1 cup	60
tangerine	115
watermelon, 6" x ½" slice	90

Vegetables

There are two vegetable lists. List A contains vegetables that are low in calories and high in vitamins. You must have at least one serving of a vegetable from this list every day. List B contains vegetables that are mostly low in calories but do not contain vitamins that are as essential as those on the A list. Some of these vegetables, however, such as peas and artichokes, are actually rather high in calories and should not be eaten too frequently if you are trying to lose weight. The low-calorie vegetables on this list are very good filler foods.

LIST A

beans, green, ½ cup	20
broccoli, ½ cup	25
cabbage, ½ cup	12
carrots, 1 cup	40
chicory, 20 leaves	10
escarole, 2 large leaves	8
kale, ½ cup	15
okra, ½ cup	35
pepper, green	15
potato, baked or boiled, small	80

spinach, ½ cup	20
squash, acorn, ½ cup	70
tomato, raw, medium	30

LIST B

artichoke, medium	50
asparagus, ½ cup	35
bean sprouts, ½ cup	12
beans, wax, ½ cup	20
beets, ½ cup	28
Brussels sprouts, ½ cup	30
cauliflower, ½ cup	15
celery, 1 large stalk	10
cucumber, medium	30
eggplant, 2 ½-inch slices	30
leek	10
lettuce, iceberg, ¼ head	15
mushrooms, ½ cup	15
onions, ½ cup	35
peas, ½ cup	60
radishes, 5	10
romaine, 5 leaves	10
scallions, 4	15
turnip, ½ cup	18
yellow squash, ½ cup	15
zucchini, ½ cup	15

Grains

brown bread, 1 slice	100
cracked wheat bread, 1 slice	60
diet bread, 1 slice	60
dry cereal, 1 ounce	110
French, Italian, or Vienna bread 1 slice, 1 inch thick	55
granola, 1 ounce	135
hard roll	160
macaroni, elbow, cooked, ½ cup	100

muffin, bran	105
muffin, corn	200
muffin, plain	140
noodles, cooked, ½ cup	100
raisin bread, 1 slice	65
rice, instant, cooked, ½ cup	75
rice, long grain, cooked, ½ cup	90
rye bread, 1 slice	70
soft dinner roll	100
spaghetti, cooked, 1 cup	155
white bread, 1 slice	65
whole wheat bread, 1 slice	60
whole wheat roll	100

Dairy Products

butter, 1 tablespoon	100
buttermilk, 8 ounces	90
egg, boiled or poached	75
egg, fried in butter	110
egg, scrambled in butter	110
milk, whole, 8 ounces	160
milk, skim, 8 ounces	90

CHEESE

American, 2 slices	210
blue or roquefort, 1 ounce	100
cheddar, 1 slice	105
colby, 1 ounce	110
cottage, ½ cup	120
edam, 1 ounce	100
gouda, 1 ounce	85
muenster, 1 ounce	100
parmesan or romano, 1 tablespoon	25

Protein Foods

BEEF

club steak, 4 ounces	335
corned beef, medium slice	240
corned beef hash, 1 cup	290
flank steak, small slice	250
hamburger, 4 ounces	220
London broil, small slice	250
porterhouse steak, broiled, medium	270
pot pie, beef, frozen	445
rib roast, medium slice	150
sirloin steak, medium	240
sirloin tip roast, medium slice	230

VARIETY MEATS

kidneys, veal, 2 small	200
liver, calf's, broiled, 3 small pieces	280

POULTRY

chicken, boned, cooked, diced, 1/4 cup	120
chicken, broiled, poached, or roasted, medium slice	110
chicken pot pie, frozen	500
turkey, roast, medium slice	100

SEAFOOD

bass, baked, medium	280
bluefish, broiled, medium	180
butterfish, fried, medium	200
clams, 10	80
cod steak, baked, medium	165
fish sticks, 3	120
flounder or sole, baked, small portion	150
halibut, baked, 4 ounces	200
oysters, raw, 6	85
salmon steak, baked, medium	180

scallops, poached or boiled, 4 ounces   80
shrimp, boiled or canned, 10 medium   120
whitefish, baked or poached, 4 ounces   210

LAMB
chop, broiled, large   145
patty, ground, 4 ounces   200
leg, roast, small slice   210

PORK
bacon, 4 strips   200
Canadian bacon, 1 slice   75
ham, smoked, 1 small slice   150
shoulder butt, medium slice   300

VEAL
cutlet, breaded and fried, small   280
leg or shoulder, roast, small slice   85
loin chop, broiled, small   180

LUNCHEON MEATS
bologna, 3 slices   140
ham, boiled, 2 slices   160
hot dog   155
liverwurst, 2 slices   150
Polish sausage, 2 inches   150
salami, 2 slices   140
Vienna sausage, 3   125

A Word of Warning about Diet Pills

Taking diet pills, or amphetamines, looks like an easy way to diet. You swallow a pill and, magically, your appetite seems to disappear. For anyone who has ever suffered hunger pangs or the pain of trying to diet when you are really hungry, diet pills sound too good to be true. But they have definite drawbacks that apply to both adults and teens.

First, diet pills do not change your eating habits. The glutton still lives in you, and when you go off the pills, as you must do if you are not to become addicted to them, you will resume your old eating habits. And you will regain any lost weight and maybe some extra to boot.

Diet pills also often have unpleasant side effects. The most serious is the possibility that you may become addicted to the pills. Other side effects include flightiness, nervousness, and an upset stomach. In addition, sometimes having no appetite is as wearing on you as having too much.

Obviously, diet pills will be available to you if you want them, but they are not a long-term answer to an overeating problem. Changing your eating habits is a much more effective, safe, and sensible way to deal with the problem of overeating. And it will be easier to develop new eating habits now while you are a teen than when you are older and more settled in your ways.

Brown-Bagging with Diet Foods

A school lunch is the perfect time to cop out on a diet. You promise yourself you will diet your way through the cafeteria line—after all, there are all those dishes of cottage cheese and fruit, so how can you miss? Easy. You go right past all the good diet foods and head for a half-pint of milk and chocolate cake. In one simple stroke, you have blown your diet—for one day, at least.

The only safe way to diet your way through a school cafe-

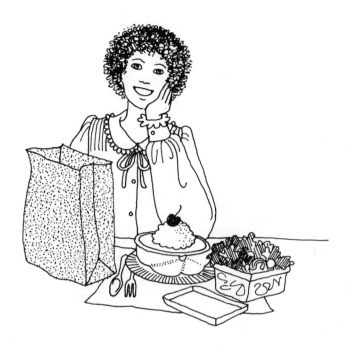

teria line is not to go through it. Instead, pack your lunch. At most, buy some milk at school—and if you are feeling especially weak one day, ask a friend to get you some when she goes through the line. Here are some suggestions for low-calorie foods to tuck away in your brown bag:

chef's salad (lettuce, tomato, cucumber, and ham or chicken)
small dinner roll
orange

⇛ ⇛

egg salad sandwich on 1 slice whole wheat bread
apple
milk

❧ ❧

2 deviled eggs
2 small tangerines
milk

❧ ❧

half melon
¾ cup cottage cheese
small green salad

❧ ❧

1 ounce hard cheese (Swiss, cheddar)
large green salad
apple
milk

❧ ❧

10 boiled shrimp
1 cup bouillon
pear
milk

❧ ❧

chicken leg and thigh
small green salad
small dinner roll with 1 teaspoon butter

These low-calorie lunches are not strictly diet lunches. If you are on a strict diet, you should pack exactly what that diet calls for rather than one of these lunches. A few weeks of these lunches will, however, help you to take off a couple of pounds.

Finally, give yourself a midafternoon snack, especially if this is the time of day when you feel your energy waning. Going to school is hard work, and if you think you need a midafternoon pick-me-up, then you probably do. Have an apple or other piece of fruit, or treat yourself to a large bowl of vegetables such as carrots, tomatoes, and cauliflower or celery. A 1½-ounce box of raisins also makes a good snack.

Eating Out When You are Dieting

It is hard to turn down dinner invitations just because you are dieting, and if you master a little restraint, this won't be necessary.

Eating out does mean that you will be faced with an array of foods—mostly forbidden foods. There are some solutions to this dilemma:

• If possible, opt for a Chinese restaurant. You just can't do much damage to your diet in one. Sauces are minimal and the foods, with little meat and many vegetables, are low-calorie. Skip noodle and other starch dishes; eat only a small portion of rice, if you must.

• As good as Chinese food can be for a diet, that's how bad Italian food can be. However, you may not have a choice over whether or not to eat in an Italian restaurant. And with care, you can still manage to be a cautious eater. First, do not even read the pasta column of the menu. Instead, go directly to the veal and poultry and order some—*without* sauce. Add a green salad, dressed lightly with vinegar and maybe some oil, and some fruit for dessert, and you have managed to eat a fairly low-calorie Italian meal.

• In other restaurants, develop an eye for low-calorie foods. Order a glass of juice or a shrimp cocktail for an appetizer. Order clear soups instead of cream-based ones. Choose a roasted or broiled piece of meat or chicken for your main course, and accompany this with a green salad, again dressed with a light portion of vinegar and oil.

• Bad diet foods to order in restaurants include anything in a rich cream sauce, anything fried, and creamy salad dressings. Don't order starches: breads, rolls, pasta, macaroni, noodles, spaetzle. Try to cut out desserts altogether. If you simply cannot manage this, settle on a piece of melon or a small dish of sherbet.

• Decline any offer of a doggie bag. No matter how good the meal, tomorrow it's back to the strict diet. And a doggie bag sitting in the refrigerator will only tempt you into letting your diet lapse for another meal.

• Finally, don't talk about your diet. Everyone talks about diets all the time, to the point where it has become an old subject. And how will a friend who is dying to order pasta feel when you start talking about what you may or may not eat? It just isn't good manners to discuss your diet anymore.

Foods for Snacks

There will be times when you will simply have to eat something that isn't part of your daily planned menu. You are starving, and if you don't nibble on something, you will lose all control and go on an eating binge. So before you get to the binge stage, treat yourself to one of these low-calorie snacks. If necessary, go on a binge eating *these* foods. You will consume some extra calories, but not as many as if you succumbed to a soda or a malted milk.

Eat-All-You-Want Foods	Good Snack Foods in Small Quantities
carrots	apple
cauliflower	melon, ½
celery	tomato
cucumber	bouillon, 8 ounces
green pepper rings	tomato juice, 8 ounces
radishes	skim milk, 8 ounces

Positively Sinful Snack Foods

Here are the foods that can really hurt. Of course, one chocolate kiss, you may note, or one walnut, does not contain many calories—but whoever heard of eating just one of these?

bread pudding with raisins	315
chocolate cupcake with icing	285
eclair	325
strawberry shortcake with whipped cream	400
piece of pie	300
chocolate cookie	100
10 walnuts	200
banana split	680
soda	250
malted milk, 8 ounces	500
milk shake, 8 ounces	420
5 caramels	400
5 chocolate kisses	100

Hints to Help You Diet

• Pick a reasonable goal. Plan to lose ten pounds in one month. If you need to lose more weight, set several goals for yourself and work toward them one at a time.

When you know that a period of tension in your life is coming up—one in which you will want to turn to food—prepare a large batch of low-calorie snacks for the dangerous moments of temptation.

• Pull a Scarlett O'Hara before parties. Mammy used to make her eat a full meal *before* she went to a party so she would "eat like a bird" and appear dainty in public. If you know you are going to a party where you will be tempted by a lot of fattening foods, eat a lot of filling, low-calorie snacks before you go so you won't be so hungry and tempted to go off your diet.

• Try to keep your life in balance when you are dieting. Dieting does throw your life off a little bit, so this is a time to be kind to yourself in other areas—get enough sleep and lots of exercise.

• Splurge once in a while. You are, after all, only human, and the craving for a piece of pie or a sundae won't vanish just because you are dieting. Rather than wait for an uncontrollable binge to come along, allow yourself a preplanned little one every so often.

• Plan a reward when you have reached your goal. Yes, losing weight is a reward in itself, but buying a new skirt in a smaller size will make it all seem even more worthwhile.

CLOTHES MAKE THE TEEN

≈§ What you wear tells a lot about you. Are you, for example, the tailored, somewhat scholarly type who prefers tweed and plaid skirts or pants with plain sweaters? Are you the outgoing type who loves to wear bright colors? Are you the creative type, favoring loose, colorful blouses and black pants or tights with skirts? Are jeans your very favorite item of clothing? Or do you prefer a flowery tie blouse with a pale-colored skirt? Your clothes probably already show signs of your personal style.

Developing a Personal Style

Perhaps the hardest part of learning how to dress involves developing a style that is exactly right for you—a style that *is* you. Some women do not manage to do this until they are in their twenties or thirties, and some women never do. The latter kind of women usually become slaves to fashion—wearing whatever is "in" at the minute whether or not it looks good on them—or they disregard fashion altogether and wear only "safe" and slightly boring clothes.

Your teen years are years of experimentation—a time when you can try lots of different looks to see what suits you and your personality. Obviously, you may not want or be able to wear completely different looks every day, but you can have variety—a ruffly blouse to suit your frilly moods and jeans and tailored shirts for casual occasions. Gradually, you will find yourself becoming more comfortable in some kinds of clothes than in others—and this style, cultivated and polished by you, will become your own individual fashion look.

Dressing for Your Age

Too many teens make the mistake of overdressing or trying to look older than they are. It is rarely successful. Understandably, you are no longer interested in wearing girlish clothes, but clothes that are too old for you are not the answer. One teen model we know solves this problem by wearing plain skirts, sweaters, blouses, and shirts—these are clothes that have no age. Another smart teen carefully reads the fashion magazines—and then chooses from the new fashion looks her own highly personal yet pulled-together style.

Dressing to Suit Your Figure

Your body shape is the single most important consideration when you are choosing clothes. Too often, teens and even older women are concerned only with hiding certain figure flaws, when, in fact, it is important also to learn to enhance your figure—to wear clothes and colors that show you off to your best advantage.

Here is a rundown of the basic figure types. Which one comes closest to describing you?

Average. If you have an average figure, everything is pretty much in proportion. Not only do you not weigh too much or too little, but your shoulders are not too broad or too round. You can wear clothes without having to make any alterations in them. Most clothes look good on you. You are very lucky—

and you are also quite rare. Even models do not fall into the average range—they are usually taller and skinnier than the average woman.

Hourglass or Slightly Heavy. This figure type ranges from the person who merely has a lot of nice curves to the person who is slightly or even drastically overweight. If you are drastically overweight (more than 10 percent above the suggested weight for your height as shown in the chart in Chapter 10), what you need to do is lose weight. You may have read that you should wear dark colors and avoid large prints and plaids, but the sad fact is that if you weigh thirty or forty pounds too much, there is little you can do in the way of dress to make yourself look smaller. Your best bet is to dress tastefully and diet and exercise to lose those extra pounds.

Teens who are only slightly overweight or who have rounded figures need to take extra care to buy clothes that fit well. Clothes should not be too tight or too loose—neither will particularly flatter you. If you are also short, you may want to avoid large plaids or prints. They will be overpowering. Go for a simple look—flared skirts, tailored pants, simple sweaters. Avoid excessive frills, outrageous styles, and shiny fabrics, all of which will make you look larger than you are. Don't wear pleated skirts or pants. Full-sleeved blouses are a good camouflage for heavy upper arms.

Short. If you are unusually short, your clothes need to be in perfect proportion.

Watch your hem lengths. You need to find the best length for you and stay with it. If skirts are a little longer one year, you may want to buy yours slightly longer but not quite as long as fashion dictates.

Miniskirts also make a short person look all chopped up, so if these return to style, you may want to go shorter but not quite as short as style dictates.

Short teens often choose very high heels on the theory that they will make them look taller. What they make you look is badly out of proportion and silly. However stylish, high heels probably aren't worth it in terms of what they do to your overall length. They are also not good for your back. Choose low to medium heel heights for a good, proportioned look.

You can carry a big purse if you like, but it probably shouldn't be as large as the big purse that a taller person would choose.

Wear single-color outfits and coordinated outfits in one color family.

Develop an eye for small details—little pockets, small collars, narrow waistbands. All these help to keep short persons in proportion. Jackets and vests should be fairly short and hit you at just the right length or you will look dumpy. Finally, look for long lines in skirts and dresses—long side openings or pleats or lengthwise stitching.

Tall. You can carry off large plaids and prints, and the soft look is perfect for you. In fact, tall teens should be careful to avoid an overly severe, too-tailored look. A close-fitting turtleneck and tailored pants, for example, are probably too severe for you. Instead, choose a full skirt, a soft tie or ruffled blouse, and a bulky cardigan sweater. Gathered or pleated skirts, soft blouses, pleated pants, and bulky sweaters are all just right for you. You can also wear contrasting colors (a green skirt and a gray blazer, for example) to break up your height, whereas a shorter person is better off sticking to one color.

Slender. If you think you are too skinny, you can dress to minimize this look. In fact, there are two tacks you can take to make yourself look fuller. First, if you are tall enough, you can wear almost anything just recommended for tall teens. If you aren't very tall, go for a layered look instead. Wear a blouse with a tie at the neckline, covered by a sweater, and then add a jacket or blazer. The lean, tailored look without layering is probably too severe for you and will only make you look even more slender.

Teens worry a lot about the size of their breasts. Almost no one thinks she has perfectly sized ones—they are invariably

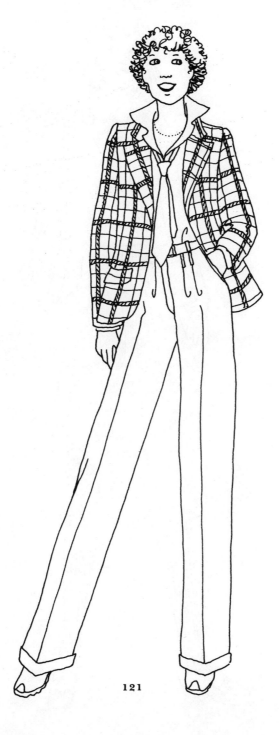

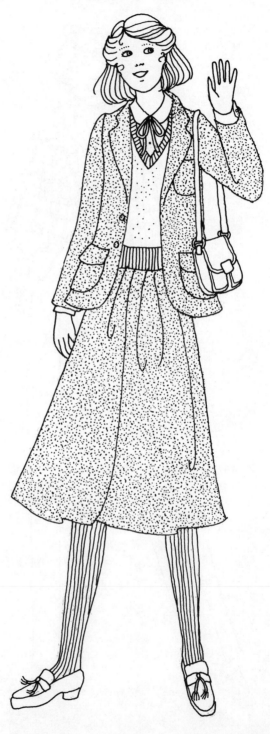

seen as either too large or too small. So here is some advice on how to make the most of what you have or do not have.

Small Breasts. Gathered, yoked blouses or blouses with front pockets or pleats are perfect for you. Tie blouses are also good, as are fairly loose-fitting sweaters. Snugly-fitting sweaters and tailored shirts will probably only emphasize your small breasts.

Large Breasts. Vertical lines are good for you—a V-necked shirt, for example, is especially flattering. Avoid wide belts and double-breasted jackets, as well as tight sweaters or blouses with horizontal stripes. Tie blouses and bulky sweaters, if you are not very short, may look especially good on you. Ruffles or a scarf near your face will help to focus attention on your face instead of your chest.

Finally, keep in mind that small breasts *and* large breasts are just another feature of your body. They alone don't make you unattractive or attractive. If you are comfortable with whatever size breasts you have, there is no reason to dress to accommodate them at all.

Your Face Shape and Clothes

In addition to your body shape, your face shape also affects the style of clothing that will look good on you. This is especially true if you have a long or rounded face.

Long Face. Strive for a look that makes your face look softer—cowl sweaters, ruffled sweaters or blouses, and Peter Pan collars are your look.

Round Face. Seek V-necks, long necklaces, and vertical lines, all of which will call attention downward and make your face look longer than it is. Avoid chokers and Peter Pan collars, as they will only emphasize your roundness.

These are the two general face shapes that can look different according to what you wear. Some of these guidelines may work for you, some may not make you look much different. Mostly, you have to experiment to find out what flatters you.

How to Buy Within Your Clothes Budget

Few of us have unlimited sums of money to spend on clothes —or anything, for that matter. But this need not affect how we look. French women, known the world over for their chic style of dressing, rarely have the large number of clothes American women do. Instead, they buy a few good skirts, pants, and tops and then mix and match them. This way, they appear to have lots of outfits and looks.

You can also save money by sewing all or part of your wardrobe if you are handy with a sewing machine. One teen we know has a perfectly fitted pants pattern that she uses over and over again.

Mixing and matching clothes is another way to save money. Whenever you buy an outfit, for example, never assume that the individual pieces must always be worn together. In fact, before you buy, consider how each of the pieces will go with the clothes you already own. Are you buying a pants suit of gray wool? What sweaters can you wear with the pants? How many skirts and pants can be coordinated with the gray jacket? By thinking along these lines, you will soon discover that you can take a few pieces of clothing and stretch them into several different outfits, and with the help of accessories, several different looks. Coordination is the basic rule of budgeting. If you draw up a list like the one at the end of this chapter, it might help you find ways to coordinate the clothes you own.

Another way to stretch your clothing dollars is to learn to mix inexpensive and expensive clothes. For example, shirts you plan to wear under sweaters need not be expensive. One high-fashion model even buys her shirts in the little boys' department and pays very little for them. Accessories need more originality than they do dollars, and you can always shop the basements of major department stores and budget chain stores, as well as the five and dime, to find scarves, belts, socks, purses, and other accessories. Some of the best-dressed models in the business spend lots of money on one or two wonderful pieces of clothing, then budget-shop for filler pieces.

Another trick is to buy clothes made in materials that can be worn through several seasons. Blue jeans of a medium-weight denim, for example, can be worn year round. Certain knits, gabardine, and challis can also be worn most of the year. Lightweight wools work from fall to late spring, whereas heavyweight wools are mostly worn only during the coldest winter months.

Avoid buying the very latest trends if your clothes budget is tight. Or shop around for a cheap version of this year's fad. If a beige linen vest is the item to own this year, but you suspect that it will be passé by spring of next year, why spend a lot of money on one? Also, you only need to buy a couple of hot clothing items each season to look as if you are dressed in the latest style. Just coordinate them with your basic wardrobe. The person who dresses in nothing but the latest fads may, in fact, be a little afraid of her own taste—she can only rely on what others tell her she should be wearing rather than on her judgment of what looks best on her.

Finally, don't be a snob about expensive labels. If a designer blouse originally sells for $115, a middle-priced manufacturer may well copy it and sell it for $55, and someone else will produce still another copy for $20. If you don't care about labels, and if the $20 copy is made well, this is what you want to buy. And a $20 blouse will also tend to look better than it is if you wear it with a very nicely tailored, fairly expensive skirt. This is how you can get more for your money by not letting yourself be swayed by labels.

Penny Pinchers' Guide to Determining Quality

Buying inexpensive clothing does require that you develop an eye for quality construction. Here are some hints for telling whether or not something is well-made:

• Look at the seams and the hem. The hem should be at least two inches deep, and the seams should be large enough so they won't pull apart easily. (Inexpensive garments always have smaller seam allowances than expensive garments do, so you should plan to buy an inexpensive garment a little larger than you normally would.)

- Study the stitching on the garment. Is it evenly sewn? Are loose threads trimmed away?
- Does the garment pucker or pull anywhere? Are the sleeves set into the shoulder smoothly?
- Do the pockets and any extra tailoring details lie flat?
- Do the plaids match at the seams?
- Does the zipper lie flat? Is it straight?

Penny Pinchers' Guide to Wise Shopping

- Look for clothes in unusual places. Buy a leotard for a bathing suit or look for an evening dress in the lingerie department.
- Buy off-season and shop the sales. Coats are considerably cheaper during the summer sales or at the traditional Columbus Day coat sales. Lingerie is often a good buy right after Christmas.
- Organize your shopping trips so you know what you are looking for and where you can expect to find it.
- Shop alone once you have learned how to shop. You may want to take your mother or a favorite aunt along the first few times you make major clothing purchases, but once you have begun to develop a style and know how to shop wisely, go it alone.
- Avoid compulsive buys. If you spot something unusual on sale and just have to have it, go buy yourself a cola and think it over for a few minutes.
- Don't let a salesperson talk you into something you don't want. Beware of salespeople who say everything looks good on you. Say you don't need any help until you have located what you want to try on, and then, if you feel you are easily swayed, tell the person helping you that you would prefer to try on the clothes in private. That way, you'll have some time to yourself to decide whether or not you like the item.
- Always think about what an item goes with and how good

it looks on you before you buy it. Don't get carried away and buy on impulse.

Finding Your Best Colors

Your skin tone is the most important factor in selecting colors you can wear well. You may also find that you look good in a color that matches your hair or your eyes. If you love a color that doesn't love you or look good right next to your face, you can still wear it. Just wear another color scarf near your face when you wear that color.

The colors you wear should also be geared to your personality, although this is probably something that will happen naturally. After all, we all react to colors—they make us feel good or not so good when we wear them. If you don't believe that color affects how you feel, look around you on a rainy day. Except for one or two smart people who reach for a red dress or sweater, most tend to pull drab-colored clothes out of their closets on rainy days.

The best way to learn what colors suit you is to try on a lot of colors when you are shopping. Wear little makeup and look carefully at your face when you are wearing a new color. Other people are also sensitive to colors, and if several people tell you that you look wonderful in pale yellow, chances are that it is truly a good color for you. Here is a general list of skin tones and the colors that go well with them:

Skin Tone/Hair	Complementary Colors
pale to pink skin blonde hair	beige (if skin is not too pale), violet, mauve, navy, blue, green, peach
dark skin blonde to light brown hair	burnt orange and rust, red, gold, bright blue, beige, army green, brown, peach

fair to rosy skin red hair	pink, violet, purple, navy, bright and pastel blue, white, gray, black
dark or olive skin red hair	brown, apricot, beige and light brown, rust, deep brown
fair skin brown to black hair	blue, white, yellow to gold, red, mauve, purple, navy, bright and pastel blue, gray
dark skin brown to black hair	bright colors—turquoise, bright green, raspberry and other purples and pinks

Another thing to consider when choosing colors is building your wardrobe around two or three basic colors so that you can easily mix and match your clothes. Certain colors are considered neutral because they go so well with so many other colors. These include black, which most teens would do well to avoid in large doses, red, camel, navy, gray, and beige.

Choosing the Clothes You Wear

Now that we have discussed a lot of general advice about clothes, it is time to talk specifically about your clothing needs and how to fill them.

The Right Underpinnings

Before you buy outer garments, you need the right underwear to wear with them. There is a great deal of variety in underwear these days. Even undershirts seem to be making a comeback, as are garter belts and the truly old-fashioned chemises. Most teens need several bras (some for everyday wear and some for special occasions), underpants, a couple of slips, and possibly a girdle.

Lingerie is sold in major department stores and in specialty stores. It comes in a wide price range, and you need not buy expensive underwear to have it fit you well or be nicely made. Underwear gets more expensive according to the materials it is made of—silk underpants, for example, cost more than those made of cotton. The amount of lace trim or handwork also affects the price.

Saleswomen are especially trained to help fit underwear such as bras and girdles, and their knowledge is worth taking advantage of. Don't worry about feeling shy trying on a bra in front of someone—if she is really tactful, she will probably leave you alone, returning only after you have put on the bra to help you decide how it fits.

Buying a Bra. You should never buy a bra without first trying it on to make sure that it fits properly and is comfortable. Bras are measured in two ways: the size you are around your rib cage and the cup size. Some stretch bras may not have a cup size and may only come in small, medium, or large.

The smallest bra size is 28 inches (around), and the largest is 40 or 42, depending upon the manufacturer. Cup sizes range from A to D, with A being the smallest size. The size bra you require will vary depending upon the manufacturer and the design of the bra.

Bras also come with underwires for girls with heavy breasts that need extra support, in a variety of materials and styles, and with padding.

If you feel you need a little extra padding, that is easy to come by these days. Lightly padded bras look and feel very natural, and there is no reason to think twice about buying a padded bra if you want one.

There are strapless bras for evening wear, halter bras to wear with halter-top dresses, and various other low-cut bras. For everyday wear and for sports, you need a well-made, fairly plain bra. Describe your needs to the saleswoman and ask to see a selection of bras that you may try on.

Never try on a bra over another bra. Slip on the new bra

and lean over and shake into it to fill up the cups. Stand up and pull the bra down on your rib cage so it feels comfortable. Adjust the straps if necessary.

Here is how to tell if a bra fits you well:

• The cups should fit smoothly over the breasts, with no overhang on top.

• Your breasts should be separated and fit in the cups.

• The bra should not feel tight anywhere, especially around your rib cage.

While you are trying on a bra, move around, sit down—check carefully to be sure it feels comfortable. Often, letting a saleswoman take a look at this point will help her bring you a style of bra that is exactly right for you. She is trained to spot your fitting problems.

If you find a bra you like, consider buying several of the same kind at one time.

Buying Underpants. Except for a few pretty synthetic pairs, buy cotton underpants or underpants with a cotton crotch. Always try on underpants over your regular panties. Underpants come in junior and misses sizes; junior sizes provide the best fit for teens. If you aren't sure what size you wear, tell the saleswoman your hip measurement and let her suggest the correct size. Like bras, underpants should not in any way be uncomfortable.

Buying a Girdle. In these days of women's liberation, girdles have been rather unpopular, but if you feel self-conscious about your weight, you may want to try wearing one. Girdles, which used to be heavy and constraining garments, are now made of lightweight material and can provide all degrees of control.

There are several kinds of girdles, but most teens will either need a brief, which is a short, light girdle shaped like a panty, or a pantygirdle, which usually has a longer leg than a brief does. The size girdle you buy will vary with the style and manufacturer, so go prepared to buy what fits and serves your needs.

Girdles come in hip sizes: petite, 34 inches and under; small, 34–37 inches; medium, 37–40 inches; and large, 40–44 inches. They are also made with panels to control the places where you bulge most. If you have a little too much stomach, buy a girdle with a front panel; thigh bulges call for one with side panels; for a rear end that is too prominent, choose one with back panels.

Choosing Slips. Styles in slips come and go. Some years everyone wears them; other years they are worn hardly at all. The important thing to remember is to wear a slip when you need one—that is, when you are wearing a clingy or see-through fabric. You can buy half-slips, full slips, slips with matching camisole tops, and slips with bras sewn in.

Since underwear does not show, it can be your secret personality. You may walk around in tailored tweeds and wool sweaters covering the frilliest, most feminine underwear imaginable. Do, however, give some thought to matching underwear colors to your outer garments. Beige bras and slips, for example, look better than white ones under almost everything— they show less. And dark underwear is usually necessary under dark clothing.

Outer Wear

Although you need not have separate wardrobes for all occasions, you will need some clothes for school, some for sports and other casual activities, and others for dressy occasions, plus one or two coats and jackets for cold-weather wear.

What you wear most of the time will probably be influenced by what your friends wear—the urge to look like everyone else is never stronger than during your teen years. If jeans are what most people are wearing to school, that is undoubtedly what you will wear; if skirts and nice pants are accepted, you'll probably opt for them.

The list that follows shows a basic teenage wardrobe—one that can be mixed and matched to produce many interesting outfits. There are lots of ways you can vary this, and you might want to add a few fad items every so often, but this is the basic wardrobe you need to be prepared to go anywhere and look great.

Basic Wardrobe

Here are the basics that will combine to make an interesting wardrobe. Brown is the basic color this wardrobe is built around, but you can choose any colors that suit you. As you can see, the brown tweed blazer goes well with the brown skirt, and the sweaters should all be in colors that will coordinate with the brown skirt and the pleated blue and brown skirt. Study the wardrobe carefully and you will see the numerous combinations of clothes it allows.

3 coats	raincoat
	winter dress coat (brown or gray)
	parka, down-filled
2 jackets	brown tweed blazer
	black velvet blazer
4 sweaters	beige cowlneck
	blue turtleneck
	off-white crewneck
	blue vest
2 skirts	brown gabardine
	blue and brown plaid, pleated
4 pants	2 pairs of jeans
	brown gabardine
	gray gabardine
1 dress	shirtwaist
dressy clothes	long red velvet skirt
4 blouses	white crepe tie-neck
	beige tailored silk shirt
	2 print blouses, one to go with brown outfits
	and one to go with gray outfits

12

ADDING THE FINISHING
TOUCHES

◆§ Accessories are the little details—scarves, belts, shoes, and purses, among other things—that pull an outfit together and make it look spectacular. They are the creative touches that you bring to your clothes—the personal statements you make about what you are wearing. Accessories are usually also small enough so they don't put a dent in your wallet—and this chapter contains suggestions for ways to accessorize cheaply.

Shoes

Shoes and boots are the first thing you need to coordinate with your clothes. The shoes you wear are probably mostly casual—they are worn for school, informal social occasions, and for sports. You may also find that you need a pair of shoes for dress occasions. Styles in shoes change fairly rapidly, so you may want to check out what's being worn in the fashion magazines before you go shopping. Buy whatever is in style at the moment, but keep in mind that it's important to be comfortable, and that if you buy on the conservative side, you can still look stylish and also wear a pair of shoes for a longer time.

If you can only buy one pair of dressy shoes, consider a neutral-colored (camel, navy, black, or brown), medium-heeled pump or slingback that will go with everything. If you can spring for a second pair of dressy shoes, a great-looking pair of sandals is a good second choice.

Darker colors such as black, navy, and brown are often worn in the winter, whereas beige and white are summer shoe colors. A light taupe or camel shoe can be worn all year and may be an especially good investment for this reason.

Buy the best shoes you can afford and be sure that they fit. Allow about ½ to 1 inch of space between your toe and the tip of the shoe when you are standing up. Walk around in a pair of shoes for a few minutes before you buy them, and even if you love the style, do not buy shoes that are uncomfortable. A good time to shop for shoes is late afternoon when you have been on your feet most of the day—your feet will have swollen slightly, so whatever shoes you buy will be comfortable on your feet whenever you wear them.

You will also need one or two pairs of boots—a good leather pair if you can afford them, and a rubberized pair for rainy days. Buy the leather boots in a good basic color that will go with your winter coat and many of your clothes. Your rainboots can be any color—the brighter the better for those rainy days.

Purses

Purses are like shoes in that styles change fairly quickly, and you will undoubtedly want to buy whatever is in style at the moment. Here are a few general hints on buying purses.

When buying good purses (to go with your dressy shoes, for example), buy the best you can afford. Leather is nice, but there are also some attractive purses made from synthetic materials that resemble leather. Before you buy, look carefully at how the purse is made—whether it has a nice-looking lining, whether the stitching is neatly done, how "good" the hardware looks. Perfectly matched purses and shoes are not stylish; if you can afford to, you should start a collection of purses and shoes in complementary colors. Your best bet is to coordinate at least some of your shoes and purses with your winter coat.

When buying a good leather purse, you will get more wear out of it if you buy a conservative, plain style in a basic color.

Generally, you will need a good purse—perhaps a clutch style—to go with your dressy shoes; an evening purse—perhaps made of faille, satin, or beads—and an everyday purse or book bag. If you like, a nice straw purse looks good and goes well with summer clothes.

Jewelry

Most young girls do not wear much jewelry until they become teens, and then it is hard to know what looks right. Since your teen years are a time for experimentation and a time to develop your own sense of style, you may want to try many combinations and styles of jewelry until you find what is right for you. You may even decide that you are most comfortable wearing little or no jewelry. Some beautifully dressed women who could afford to put anything they want on their backs as well as to wear any jewels they choose prefer to wear no jewelry. This is simply their look. If you have never worn jewelry, you may want to play around with wearing some before you decide to give it all up.

As a general rule, wear a little less jewelry than you think you need. No one ever says, "She is wearing too little jewelry," but people do comment about wearing too *much*.

There are different kinds of jewelry. There is, for example, real jewelry and costume jewelry. Real jewelry, which is expensive, is made from real gold and silver and precious or semiprecious stones. Costume jewelry, often made to look like real jewelry, is less expensive and is probably what you can afford to buy.

You need not spend a lot of money on jewelry—and you also need not buy only traditional jewelry. One smart teen haunts her local hardware store and often makes interesting pieces of jewelry from her finds there. The notions or ribbon section of your local department or sewing goods store sells many materials that can be converted to jewelry. Look for beads, buttons, ribbons, and other such things, with an eye for how they could be made into an interesting piece of jewelry.

There is also a difference between the kind of jewelry that is worn at night and the kind that is worn during the day. Generally, daytime jewelry is quieter, whereas evening jewelry is more likely to be glittery—made of rhinestones, or diamonds, if you please. Save your glittery jewelry for fancy dress nights.

Scarves

Scarves are a wonderful accessory because they can be used in so many ways. You can wear a scarf tied at your neck in a number of styles, wear it on your head, around your waist, or nonchalantly tied to your purse. For not very much money, you can also build a nice collection of scarves—choose bright colors and prints in a variety of fabrics such as cotton, wool, challis, and synthetics.

How you wear scarves varies with the current fad and what you are comfortable with. Fashion magazines often show different ways of using scarves. A scarf tucked in your neckline is a good way to add color to your face or to bring out the color of your eyes.

Hats

If you live in a cold climate and walk to school, you probably need a few hats. Teens rarely wear fancy hats, so you will probably want one or two simple knitted or crocheted styles. Buy hats to go with but not necessarily match your coats or jackets. If you are planning to wear a scarf and a hat, they should go well together, but they need not match or even be made from the same material.

Gloves

Years ago, gloves were the mark of a lady, and a set of elaborate rules dictated where and how they would be worn. Today, almost everyone wears gloves mostly for warmth or to accessorize an outfit—and teens are no exception. Casual gloves come in a variety of materials, ranging from suede and leather to synthetic and knits.

Before you buy gloves, you need to know what size you wear. To determine your approximate glove size, put a tape measure around your hand at its widest point, usually just below your fingers. This figure, probably around 6 or 7 inches, is your glove size, although the actual size you wear may vary with the manufacturer and kind of glove.

Gloves are also described by button length. One-button gloves are the short, wrist-length ones you most often wear for casual occasions. Sixteen-button gloves, also called opera-length, are worn for very formal occasions—they come to the middle of your upper arm. A three- or four-button length will give you good protection from the weather if you live where winters are very cold.

When buying gloves, select them in colors that go with your coat and any hat or scarf you may wear.

Belts

Belts not only hold up jeans, but they are an important fashion accessory. In the illustrations below you can see a couple of belt styles and the moods they create. How belts are worn is generally a matter of fashion, but you can almost always get by with one or two styles. Your first investment should be a

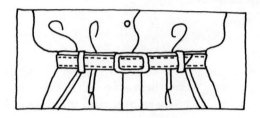

good leather belt with a plain buckle. A straw belt is also good for summer. When choosing basic belts, pick ones that will look good with jeans, skirts, and dresses, if possible.

If you buy a dress or pants suit that comes with a belt, do not fall into the trap of thinking of that belt as part of that outfit only. Pull it off and test it with your other clothes to see what it looks good with. You can also make your own belts. Materials for casual jeans belts and dressy belts for evening wear can often be found in the notions and yard goods sections of department or sewing stores. For evening wear, look for interesting silk cords that you can twist and knot into a belt. Braid trims sewn to buckles make interesting jeans and pants belts.

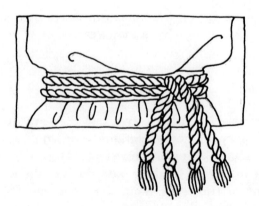

Stockings

Pantyhose are probably the mainstay of your stocking wardrobe. They can be purchased in all sizes and colors, and in plain or textured styles. Pantyhose come in small, medium, and large sizes, but their fit varies with the manufacturer, so try several pairs until you find a brand that really fits you well (without bagging anywhere and without fitting so tightly at the waist that eating is agony) and then always try to buy that brand. You'll need several pairs in neutral skin-toned colors, plus whatever you want to match with various outfits. Textured hose worn, for example, with a tweed skirt or dark-colored skirt, can really change the look of an outfit. Try to vary your pantyhose wardrobe—don't be the girl who *always* wears black tights. Also, for hygienic reasons, look for a brand with a cotton crotch if you plan to wear them without underpants.

There has been a return in recent years to regular hose worn with a garter belt, and you might find it fun to try them, although pantyhose are generally more suited to everyday use. You can also buy knee-high hose in a variety of colors and textures to wear under pants. Knee-high hose should never be worn with skirts or with any outfit where they will show—only knee socks in solid or opaque materials and pretty colors and patterns are meant to be worn this way.

Hose are not an especially durable item, and you will have to get used to tossing them out when they are no longer fit to be worn. Never wear hose with a run or hole in them, nor should they be worn if they are the slightest bit mottled-looking. Hose, especially skin-color hose, should make your legs look sleek and smooth.

Because they are so fragile, you can't just toss hose in the washing machine as you can knee socks. The amount of time they last depends upon the kind of care you give them. Chapter 13 contains information on how to take care of your hose.

Glasses

Glasses are probably your most important fashion accessory
—and they certainly are the most expensive. The best way to
find glasses that are right for you is to go to a store that sells
them and try on as many pairs as you can—until you find
the pair that looks great on you. With the great variety of
styles available today, no one needs to look unattractive in
glasses.

Prepare carefully for your shopping expedition. Make up
carefully, and make sure your hair looks nice and is in the
style in which you usually wear it.

Fashions in glasses come and go (although not as frequently
as other areas of fashion, thank heaven), and if you can't afford
to buy new ones every time the styles change slightly, your
best bet is to buy something that is stylish yet conservative.

Glasses should flatter your face shape. Here are some general
guidelines for wearing glasses to suit your face shape.

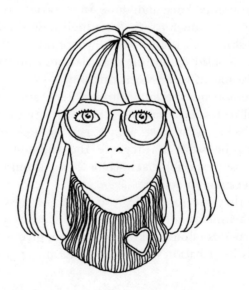

Oval Face. This perfectly shaped face can wear almost any kind of glasses.

Heart-Shaped Face. Look for a softly curved frame that is narrower than your forehead, which tends to be wide.

Diamond-Shaped Face. Rounded frames are flattering to you. They should be as wide as your cheeks, which are probably the widest part of your face.

Round Face. Look for a slightly squarish frame that adds angles to your rounded contours.

Long Face. Fairly big lenses are good for you. Look for a frame that is as wide as your face, but not wider.

Square Face. Look for a rounded frame that will soften the angles of your face.

The hints just offered are only guidelines. You may find a pair of glasses that is not supposed to look good on you that actually looks fabulous—by all means, buy them.

When you are trying on glasses and you come across a frame shape that looks pretty good on you, ask to see everything else that is similar. Sometimes even the tiniest angle may be the difference between a more flattering or a less flattering frame.

If possible, too, look at yourself wearing them in a full-length mirror.

If you are buying a plastic frame, be sure to choose a color that flatters your face. Black is usually too harsh, so if you want a dark color look for a brown or a tortoise. Pastel shades— pinks and blues—are especially flattering to your skin; pink really makes you glow. For drama, try bright red or green frames.

In addition to choosing a flattering frame color, you can also have the lenses tinted. If you have chosen a colored frame, the tint will probably coordinate with the frame. Sometimes just the merest hint of a tint is perfect—too much tint, particularly in a gray or blue, can make you look washed-out and may not look good in photographs.

If you wear prescription glasses, you will probably need a pair of sunglasses in addition to your regular ones. It is fun to choose frames that are entirely different from your everyday glasses. You can buy sunglasses that lighten for indoor wear and then darken when you walk out into the sun, but these are not very good if you live in a climate with a lot of strong sunshine—you would do better to get regularly tinted sunglasses in this instance. Gray is more effective than dark green for protecting your eyes from the sun, and heavy tints in blue and red do little to protect your eyes from the sun—they are mostly for show.

Making Up When You Wear Glasses

There is no question about it—glasses draw attention to your eyes. This means you should apply eye makeup a little more carefully than you normally might. Wear a little extra makeup on your eyes: apply an extra coat or two of mascara and use a pretty pastel shade of eye shadow on your eyelids. (Fancy, overdone shadowing shows more readily when you wear glasses, so keep this in mind when you make up.) Smudges and smears are also more obvious under glasses, so take extra care to apply your eye makeup perfectly. In addition, keep your eyebrows plucked neatly if they need it—they are more a center of attention when you wear glasses than when you don't.

Contact Lenses

In recent years, many new, exciting developments in contact lenses have made them more widely available and easier to wear. If you really dislike eyeglasses or if you have a vision problem that would be especially helped by wearing contact lenses, then they are worth the investment.

Contact lenses are more expensive than eyeglasses—how much more varies with where you live and how complicated your eye problems are. Contact lenses must be fitted by an optometrist or an ophthalmologist (a medical doctor trained in the care of the eyes).

Contact lenses can be tinted, which helps to eliminate the glare from the sun and also has the side benefit of enhancing the color of your eyes. Some models even own several pairs of contact lenses in colors completely different from their real eye color—something you might want to consider. Even better than totally changing your eye color, though, is bringing it out with a pair of contact lenses that darken it.

Playing the Accessory Game

Choosing and wearing accessories is a lot of fun, and it's a way to expand and test your fashion sense without spending a lot of money. You may not want to wear everything mentioned in this chapter—if you already know, for example, that you aren't the type for scarves, don't bother with them. On the other hand, if you have never tried them, buy one or two and experiment. Once you have found the accessories that look great on you and seem to go with your personal fashion style, collect them and think of as many interesting ways to wear them as possible.

Styles in accessories change rapidly—usually from season to season. And because they're cheap, you can probably afford to go with the very latest fad. Before you rush out and buy all new accessories, however, study the fashion magazines with an eye for what you already own. Do you really need new scarves? Or could you tie last year's scarves in a new way? How about that old rhinestone pin in your mother's jewelry box that you used to wear when you played dress-up? Isn't it right in style now? The most clever accessories are frequently recycled ones.

Here's a final word of warning, though: don't overdo accessories, especially the superfluous ones that you only wear to look prettier. One stunning scarf or one funny or unusual piece of jewelry is all you need to show you off at one time. If you wear too many things at once, no one of them will stand out.

13

TAKING CARE OF
YOUR CLOTHES

❧ Once you have chosen clothes that are right for you and right for all occasions, you need to consider how to take care of them. Clothes care may seem like a silly subject to take up an entire chapter, but how you take care of your clothes has a lot to do with the image you present to others. The most expensive outfit in the world will look all wrong if a button is missing or part of the hem has fallen—or even if there is a small tear in a seam. And clothes that are inexpensive will always look a little nicer than they are if they are carefully pressed and in good repair.

Various kinds of garments require different methods of care. Some things have to be hand-washed, for example, while others must be dry-cleaned. Some raincoats or all-weather coats are waterproofed; others must be waterproofed by your dry cleaner. Fine wools can either be washed or dry-cleaned, and there is a great difference in cost and time, as we shall see later, depending upon which method you use.

Surprisingly, the time to think about taking care of your clothes is before you buy them. That's right. Don't spend your money on yet another blouse that has to be hand-washed if you already have more blouses than you can possibly take care of. Don't buy another item in a light color that will require a lot of dry cleaning if your dry cleaning budget is already tight. You aren't really getting full wear out of a garment that hangs in your closet because it needs laundering or dry cleaning when you do not have the time or money to do either. So think before you buy: how much care will this garment require, and am I willing to take care of it properly so that I can wear it frequently?

Clothes care falls into three general categories: general maintenance, which basically means making sure that any item of clothing you pull out of your closet is clean and ready to wear; special care, the maintenance you have to do on leather shoes and boots, suedes, and brass trim, for example; and alterations, the fairly major sewing tasks that make clothes just right for your body.

Taking Care of Your Clothes

Routine care is the key to maintaining your wardrobe so that everything is ready to wear at any time. Form the habit of checking clothes before you put them away and after you have worn them. Set aside anything that needs repairing—a torn seam, a hem that has come unsewn, or a missing button are all minor repairs. Do these repairs frequently and regularly. Leaving these clothes out when they need repair will let them serve as a reminder to you that they need work. Also, you won't want to look at a pile of clothes in your bedroom for very long. Never put something away that needs repair— you'll only forget about it and be upset the next time you want to wear it.

Clothes Maintenance Supplies

You need a few supplies for regular maintenance of your clothes. If possible, keep these supplies together in a basket or some other container that you can easily carry from your bedroom to the bathroom or laundry room. Here is a list of basic supplies for maintaining your clothes:

- Cold water soap for wool and delicate clothes.
- Plastic hangers, perhaps inflatable, for drying wet clothes.
- Plastic bags for storing clean clothes.
- Clothes brushes, one for wools and others for suedes. Use one brush for light-colored suede and another for dark-colored suede.
- Spot remover for clothes that need touch-ups between dry cleanings.
- Shoe polish and anything you need for polishing your shoes (rags, brushes, etc.). Be sure to have the proper polish for every pair you own.
- Brass cleaner for coat fasteners and belt buckles.
- Jewelry cleaner.
- Sewing kit containing basic sewing supplies, and including thread to match every outfit you own. (One model we know stops at the dime store on the way home from shopping trips and buys thread and buttons to match anything she has just bought. She may not need the thread for months, but she's prepared when the day for minor repairs comes.)
- File of washing and cleaning instructions for your clothes. Whenever you buy something new, store the tags (after you have labeled them) in this file. If you want to, clip off labels and staple them to 3″ x 5″ index cards on which you have written a brief description of the article. Clothes without labels fit smoother, and your washing instructions will always be close at hand this way.

The first thing you need to do to maintain your clothes is to treat them with respect. This means hanging everything up right after you have worn it. Clothes draped over chairs even for one night lose some of their shape and almost certainly need to be pressed before you wear them. Skirts, pants, dresses, and blouses all should be hung on hangers. You can buy special hangers for these clothes, or you can use regular wire hangers. Pants should be hung on special pants hangers, wooden or plastic hangers, or on a wire hanger that has a roll of cardboard around the bottom wire—this way, they won't get a heavy crease around the knees. Better still is to hang them from the waist, as stores do. You can buy special hangers or use clothes pins or safety pins.

If an article of clothing needs pressing, do this before you put it away. Brush clothes before you put them in the closet, so that any hairs and lint that have accumulated during wear won't rub off on your other clothes.

Keeping Clothes Clean

Sort out clothes that need cleaning. Most clothes will need either dry cleaning, regular washing, or hand washing, depending on the materials they are made of.

Wool clothes need to be dry-cleaned, although you can wash your woolens by hand in a cold-water soap if you like. Special instructions on doing this are given in this chapter in the section on hand laundry. Wool sweaters and other knitted items respond best to this treatment; wool skirts and jackets are best treated to professional dry cleaning.

Most cottons can be tossed in the regular laundry or hand-washed. Read the instructions on the care label to double check.

Synthetics require a wide variety of care. Some need to be dry-cleaned; others need hand washing; and fortunately, increasing numbers can be washed with the regular laundry.

Since dry cleaning is expensive, you will probably want to do it as infrequently as possible. There are ways to save on trips to the dry cleaner. A good spot remover helps. Look over a piece of clothing each time you wear it and use the spot remover wherever necessary. Think of dry cleaning only as a means of cleaning your clothes, not as a means of pressing them. Do all your own pressing at home. The exception to this is a stained piece of clothing. Never press a stain because the hot iron tends to set it and make it harder to remove. Clothes stains that do not come out with the spot remover should be taken immediately to the dry cleaner—before you forget what caused the stain. Be sure to point out the stain and tell the cleaner what it is.

Regular Laundry

This is far and away the easiest way to launder an article of clothing. You simply separate dirty clothes into batches of white, medium-colored, and dark, and put them in a washing machine with a soap or detergent, set the dials for the type of laundering you need, and start the machine. Most teens are especially lucky in this department because their mothers do the family laundry. Yet part of taking care of your clothes well involves knowing how to do everything, so you should offer your mother a hand.

Hand Laundry

This is for special items, wool sweaters, and the other knitted items such as scarves and gloves. Hand laundry is done in a small basin using a cold-water soap. Here are a few guidelines for washing wools or delicate fabrics by hand:

1. Wash the article according to package directions in a cold-water soap designed for use on delicate materials.
2. Let the article soak exactly as long as the package directions specify; longer soaking just lets the loosened dirt settle back in.
3. Rinse the article in cold or lukewarm water. Do not squeeze or pull it; simply push it up and down in several changes of water and then let the water run over it for a few minutes. Squeeze very gently.
4. Carefully lay out the article on a heavy towel and then roll it up to remove excess moisture.
5. On a table or other drying surface, or in the bathtub,

carefully place the article on another towel. Arrange it into its regular shape and smooth it out. Let it dry naturally, away from any artificial sources of heat. (Drying a sweater over a radiator is a sure way to shrink it.)

6. If necessary, touch up the article with a warm steam iron when it is nearly dry.

7. Return it to still another towel to finish drying overnight.

Ironing and Pressing

All seamstresses know that half the art of making a piece of clothing look well-tailored is pressing it correctly as it is sewn. The same principle applies to any pressing you do on your clothes after they are sewn and in your closet. It is worthwhile taking a few minutes to learn how to press correctly for the dividends you will reap in looking neater.

You need first of all to understand an iron, your basic pressing tool. Ironing, done without steam, is heavy-duty work done on some clothes right after they have been washed. You would, for example, iron a cotton blouse as the finishing touch to cleaning it. Pressing is done with steam.

Most irons are carefully marked with the temperature for each fabric. If in doubt, set the temperature a little lower than the care instruction label recommends. When pressing wool or pressing a new hem or seam, consider using no steam, and, instead, placing a damp cotton cloth or tea towel over the item you are pressing. Place the iron gently on top of the tea towel; the steam generated by the wet towel gives a firmer press than does using a steam iron alone.

Whether pressing or ironing, do small details first and then finish with the larger sections. Here, for example, is the order in which to press the parts of a blouse (which should give you an idea of the order in which to press other items): start with the back of the collar; press the front of the collar; the yoke, if there is one; the cuffs of the sleeves; the sleeves; the front sections; and finally the rest of the back section (below the yoke). If there are pockets on the front, press them before pressing the front.

Knowing when to iron or press something should be no problem: you do so at the first sign of a wrinkle.

Special Care

Items that require special care include shoes and boots; brass trim on purses, coats, and shoes; and jewelry. Let's start with the easiest first: jewelry. Buy a jar of jewelry cleaner from your local jeweler. Usually ammonia-based, these cleansers come with a small tray or brush so you can dip the jewelry in the solution and then lightly brush to remove any extra dirt. This kind of cleaning is good only for gold and silver and other metal jewelry.

Jewelry with set stones can be lightly cleaned with the solution, but you should not dunk it for any length of time as this will tend to loosen the stones.

Costume jewelry made from other materials—ceramic, for example—should be cleaned by gently wiping with a damp cloth.

Watches, especially good ones, need periodic cleaning and checking by your jeweler. Take your watch for a regular checkup every two years or so.

Suede and leather require special cleaning attention. Both need dry cleaning of a type that is very expensive, so wear these items with great care. Brush suede after every wearing. Store suede and leather garments in garment bags when you are not wearing them.

Leather boots probably take more wear and tear than any other thing you own, but they will last a long time if given proper care between wearings. Use saddle soap every few months to keep the leather supple. You can also protect leather from bad weather by applying a water repellent several times during the winter. Choose either a silicone-based or an oil-based one. The silicone will eventually make the leather shiny, which is fine for some leathers but not for others. The oil-based repellent tends to darken leathers. Buy whichever repellent suits your boots. Leather gives and becomes more supple with age, and rubbing in repellents and oils encourages this process, so don't overdo the cleaning and protection. A few times a winter is often enough.

If you live in a northern climate that gets lots of snow, you will also need a salt repellent, which you can purchase from a shoe repair or shoe store.

Leather shoes do not necessarily need water-repellent treatments or saddle-soaping on a regular basis, although it's something to consider on shoes that you wear outside a lot in bad weather. They do, however, need regular cleaning and polishing. Use polish that matches the shoe color, and buff with a clean cloth to a soft shine.

Shoes need reheeling and resoling when these parts wear out. This is a job for a good shoe-repair person. Just be sure to take your shoes in for this treatment before they look really worn down. Shoes that badly need reheeling—or worse, shoes with worn soles—look sloppy and can ruin the look of whatever else you are wearing.

Brass trim, commonly used on shoes and purses, tarnishes if not given some care. One trick some models use is to coat new brass trim with clear nail polish to prevent tarnishing. Be careful not to get any polish on the surrounding fabric, and let the piece of clothing dry thoroughly before you wear it. Another way to maintain brass trim is to buy a special cleaner designed for use on brass. Wrap aluminum foil around the fabric under the brass trim and apply the cleaner according to package directions.

Stains on Clothing

As embarrassing as it may seem to spill something on yourself, everyone does it at one time or another. Your main concern when this happens should be to save or preserve the outfit you have stained. Immediately after spilling something, wet the stain with cold water. Most food stains, except for oils, will come out with this treatment.

Take the item to the dry cleaner as soon as possible, point out what the stain is, and ask them to pay special attention to it.

The chart that follows shows stopgap remedies you can use for common stains until you can get the clothes to the cleaner.

Stain-Removal Chart

BLOOD	Rinse washables immediately in cold water or soak in presoak or detergent. Launder as you regularly would. Rub nonwashables with a mixture of 3 tablespoons salt in a quart of water, then dry-clean.
CHEWING GUM	Scrape off as much as you can with a knife. Put the stained area between sheets of tissue paper and press with a warm iron to loosen the gum.
COFFEE	Soak washables in warm water with a presoak. Launder immediately. Nonwashables should be dry-cleaned.
CHOCOLATE	Same as coffee.
GRASS	Rub with detergent or soak in presoak for colored washables. Use water temperature recommended on presoak label. Use bleach on white washables. Dry-clean nonwashables.
GREASE	Launder or dry-clean immediately.
LIPSTICK	Use bleach on whites; launder colored clothes. Dry-clean nonwashables.
MILDEW	Launder with detergent (use water temperature suggested on label) and use bleach on white washables. Dry-clean nonwashables.
WAX	Scrape off as much as you can with a knife. Put the stained area between two absorbent surfaces (tissue works well here) and press with a warm iron.

Altering Your Clothes

Once you have learned how to maintain your clothes, the next thing to think about is alterations, those small or sometimes major sewing jobs that can change the look of an outfit.

Alterations, like regular maintenance, are something to consider before you buy. As a general rule, don't buy something that requires major alterations. If the designer of a jacket thought it would look better without epaulets, he or she would not have added them. Drastically lengthening or shortening an article of clothing is often a mistake—again, the item is designed for one length, and it will never look quite the same. It may not fit so smoothly or hang properly after a major alteration. Coats, for example, rarely can be cut off into jackets without ruining their lines. You can easily change a long skirt into a short skirt, though, and you should not hesitate to do this to give new life to an outfit.

Check your clothes periodically to be sure they are in good condition. A coat you wear every day may have frayed at the sleeves, or the lining may be torn, and you may fail to notice this simply because you wear the coat every day and have stopped "seeing" it.

Complicated alterations and repairs should be taken to a seamstress or tailor. Many dry cleaners can do basic alterations for you for a small extra charge. Complicated jobs that you should not attempt yourself unless you are a skilled seamstress include zipper repairs, waistband repairs, and shoulder repairs. You can fix hems and torn seams and linings, and sew on buttons yourself, however, and save the expense of having someone else do it.

Before you undertake minor repairs, you need to know what will work and what won't. Lengthening a garment rarely works because the old hemline always shows. It especially doesn't work on knitted clothes. Shortening, as noted earlier, works very well. Shortening a pair of pants that are too long is a simple procedure. But if pants have become too short due to changing styles, forget about lengthening them and tuck them into your boots instead.

The major repairs you will do yourself are hemming and sewing on buttons. Here are the steps to sewing a perfect hem:

1. Let down the old hem. Press it out.
2. Let someone measure where you want the new hem.
3. Attach seam binding to the raw edge of the let-down hem. (The lace seam bindings are an especially nice touch.)
4. Press the hem in place, using a damp tea towel and dry iron.
5. Sew, using a single thread and an overcast stitch (see illustration). Take small stitches and space them evenly apart. You may think that hem-stitching won't show, and it won't, but a neatly sewn hem hangs better than one done sloppily.
6. Do a final touch-up pressing.

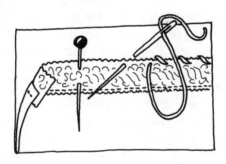

Sewing on buttons is easy enough to do haphazardly, but they will last longer and look better if you do it right. Always match the size, color, and shape of the button that is missing. It helps to keep a supply of small white and colored buttons on hand with which to repair blouses. Always match the thread, too. Use buttonhole or heavy-duty thread, or a double thread, for greater strength. Pin the button to the spot where you want

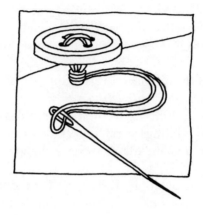

to sew it. Don't knot the thread; rather, make several tiny stitches on the underside of the fabric, which will look neater when done. Draw up the thread from underneath and sew it neatly through the holes in the button; do not sew it too tightly. As a finishing touch and for longer wear, wrap the thread around the already sewn thread (see illustration).

Sometimes a button comes off and pulls a little bit of the fabric with it. This is not a hopeless situation. Fill in with a little fabric carefully clipped from a seam allowance or facing. Sew the button on the new fabric after you have neatly and invisibly stitched the new fabric into place. Trying to sew on the button by pulling together the hole will only ensure that it will come off again—this time bringing even more fabric with it.

Emergency Repairs

Sometimes something will go wrong with a garment you are wearing after you have left home. Such incidents can be kept to a minimum by checking your clothing carefully after each wearing, but don't panic if you need to make an emergency repair.

The first step is to be prepared. Carry a small emergency repair kit with you all the time. It should contain thread (white and black or gray will do), needle, tape, safety pins, and a few blouse buttons.

If a hem comes down, sew it if possible; if too large a section has come undone, tape it until you get home. Tears in seams and other places in fabrics can be pinned, sewn, or, less often, taped. A missing button on a blouse can be quickly replaced, and other, larger buttons can be pinned on.

Another emergency that calls for action is getting caught in a storm unexpectedly. Shake out wet clothes, especially woolens, and hang them to dry in a place where the air can circulate around them freely. Do not hang them near a source of heat. When dry, brush and press them before putting away.

Stuff shoes that get wet with newspapers so they will dry in shape. Let them dry naturally, too, away from a source of heat. Clean and polish them as soon as they have dried.

Organization—the Key to Maintenance

Clothing care will be a lot easier if you are an organized person. Clothes that are properly hung in closets between wearings and stored away properly between seasons will require less maintenance. An even more important reason to keep your closets and dresser organized and clean is that you will never lose track of what you own. When you buy something new, it will be easy to pull other items of clothing to coordinate with the new outfit from a neat, well-organized closet.

There are all degrees of closet organization. You can buy many useful accessories—special hangers for pants, blouses, and skirts; padded hangers for dresses; plastic boxes to hold sweaters; hatboxes; shoe trees; and other useful items of storage. There are even sophisticated ways to rebuild closets to accommodate your needs, and if you or a friend is handy with tools, you might consider a complete overhaul. Since most teens wear so many separates, you might, for example, add a second closet pole, allowing you to hang your blouses on top and pants and skirts on the bottom. You get nearly double the usable space without actually adding any space.

If you have decided on something less than a major overhaul, there are still plenty of hints for keeping your clothes neatly organized.

- Use clear plastic bags or boxes so you can see what is in your closet.
- Label these containers so you will have yet another reminder.
- Group clothes to suit you, but have some plan. You could put all your dressy clothes in one section and all your sports clothes in another, or you could group all your blouses, all your pants, all your skirts, and so on.
- Plan to hang all your clothes except for knits.
- Buy and use some wooden or plastic hangers for coats and dresses.
- Store clothes you do not wear frequently in plastic garment bags.
- Keep sweaters and knits (neatly folded) in boxes or in dresser drawers.
- Wrap hats and purses in plastic bags to protect them when you are not using them.
- Put shoe trees in shoes that you do not wear often or store them in boxes, preferably wrapped in tissue. Store shoes you do wear often in a shoe bag.

Finally, use every single inch of space in your closet. No woman ever has enough closet space, but smart women make the most of what they have. Buy an over-the-door shoe container, or use the door for scarves and belts stored in wicker baskets that you have attached to the door. Add hooks and shelves wherever possible to make more room for your clothes.

And clean your closets regularly. Even with regular care, all closets get messy. And when closets get messy, clothing—believe it or not—gets lost. When you clean your closet, you may dis-

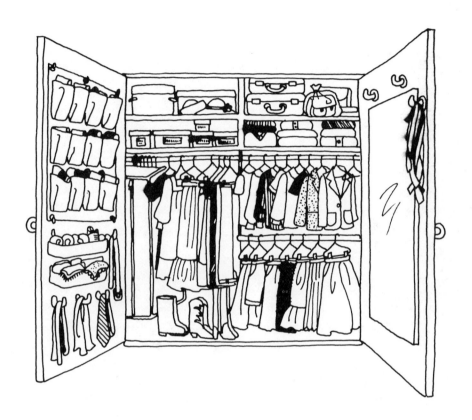

cover something that is just right to wear right now—buried on the floor.

Although there may seem to be a lot of details to clothes maintenance, it's really very easy—once you are prepared and organized for any possible situation. Maintenance should only take thirty minutes every ten days to two weeks if you are organized and ready to go when something needs doing.

14

JOB HUNTING FOR TEENS

✍§ Job hunting can be difficult. Let's face it—you are looking for part-time work, and you probably have little or no work experience. Still, finding a part-time job is not impossible, and you are ahead of the game if you know how to go about getting one.

Making the Initial Call

Once you have lined up several possible job leads, you will have to start making calls to set up appointments. If necessary, write out what you plan to say. If you are really nervous, read your statement over the telephone until you become at ease enough to speak off the top of your head. You'll sound slightly more formal reading something than if you weren't, but the person you speak with probably won't realize what you are doing.

If you are responding to an ad in the paper, you might say something such as this:

Hello, my name is Julia Jones. I'm calling about the ad you ran in Sunday's paper for a part-time veterinary assistant. I would be very interested in talking with you about the job. I love animals and have always had a pet. I feel that this is a kind of work I could do well. Could we make an appointment to talk about this further?

If you are calling a contact that someone you know has suggested to you, you might say:

Hello, my name is Susanna Taylor. My uncle, Jack Taylor of ABC Company, suggested that I call you about the possibility of part-time work. I'm wondering if you have anything available right now?
You do? That's great. Could we make an appointment to meet and discuss this more?

Both these imaginary conversations have several things in common. First, always identify yourself and tell why you are calling. Second, if possible, state very briefly why you think you might be suitable for a position. Finally, and most important, ask for an interview. Not to do so leaves things hanging in the air and defeats the entire purpose of the call.

Often, before you can get through to the person who can hire you, you will have to deal with his or her secretary or assistant. Never underestimate the influence these people have over their bosses, and always be as polite to them as you would be if you were talking to the Big Boss.

Most teens do not need a resume to interview for part-time work. (A resume is a written history of your job experience.) Sometimes, though, a simply written page outlining your job goal, your school interests and strengths, and any previous work experience may be helpful. If, for example, you are planning a heavy campaign for a summer job, such a job history, along with a very simple covering letter, might help.

A covering letter is a letter you write to introduce yourself and to ask if a job is available. You might be asked to send one if you call a business to inquire about part-time work or you might want to send a blitz of letters to a lot of prospective employers with the hope of turning up a job. Your covering letter is pretty much like a phone call: it should identify you, tell very briefly about you, and ask for an interview. You should include your address and phone number so that persons know how to contact you.

Looking Pretty for the Interview

Once you have set up an appointment, the next step is to consider how to dress for the interview. If the real you is most comfortable kicking around in jeans, that's fine, but don't give a thought to wearing them in a job interview.

One sign of being mature is recognizing that there are a few ways in which you have to conform in this world—and job hunting most certainly is one of those occasions. To add insult to injury, some adults tend to think that many teens are sloppy and poorly groomed by nature. While this isn't true—many teens today are not only neat but are style-setters as well—it's still an image you need to be aware of and to work against.

Plan to wear a fairly conservative skirt and top or pants and matching top to the interview. Whatever you wear, it should be clean and neatly pressed. Don't wear pants if you suspect that they might not be appropriate for the place where you are interviewing. A part-time job as an intern in your local bank, for example, is probably a place where a dress or skirt and top would be expected. You can undoubtedly wear pants on the job, but they aren't always a good idea for the interview.

You can wear any color you want to wear, but the style of your clothes should be fairly conservative—and this means everything you put on from head to toe. Don't wear a wild hat or the most far-out shoes you own, even if this is how you like to dress.

Check to be sure that whatever you wear is in good condition. A missing button or a tear that you failed to notice the last time you wore the outfit could cost you a job. Neatness counts to an amazing degree on a job interview. It seems to convey some idea to a prospective employer about how neatly and carefully you will do your work.

Your shoes and the purse you carry should be clean and recently polished. Check to be sure your heels are not run down, and if they are, get them repaired before the interview.

Be sure your nails are well-manicured, but wear clear or no nail polish or possibly a very pale shade of pink or peach rather than a bright color. If you are applying for a job that involves typing, make sure your nails are short enough to look as if you can actually type. Your makeup, too, should be toned down. Think about what you usually wear, then plan to wear a little less.

Jewelry should also be conservative. Wear a watch, by all means, and possibly earrings or a pin. Wear only two or three pieces of jewelry at the most, counting your watch.

Conducting the Interview

The actual interview is worrisome, perhaps because it is a reminder that you are young and inexperienced and want something from someone who is older, experienced, *and* in a position to give you what you want.

Most prospective employers will take the lead in talking, especially in the case of a teenager, so you will have little to worry about on this score.

Be sure to arrive on time or even a few minutes early for a job interview. Take into account that you may not know exactly where a place is or that you may have to wait for a slow elevator to take you to the twentieth floor—leave lots of extra time to get there.

A good trick is to arrive several minutes ahead of time and take five minutes to look yourself over in the ladies' room. Comb your hair and reapply your lipstick if necessary.

If you are interviewing with a large company or business, you will probably encounter a receptionist first. Tell the receptionist your name and whom you want to see. Mention that you have an appointment. Be sure to thank any receptionist or secretary who helps you and tell him or her good-bye when you depart.

When you enter the office of the person you are interviewing with, shake hands as you meet if you are meeting for the first time. Do not sit until you are asked to do so. Then sit up straight, but without looking overly formal. Do not lean over the person's desk or look at all curious about anything on it.

If the person is talking on the phone when you enter the room and spends a couple of minutes wrapping up the phone call, pretend you heard nothing. Even if the person goes on to comment about the phone call, saying something such as, "I was just talking to your father about our weekly golf game this Saturday," say something restrained such as, "Oh, that's nice." It may seem funny to pretend you didn't hear a conversation that went on in your presence, but it's one of those little rules of business (and sometimes social) life.

The trick to interviewing is to answer all questions honestly and still play up your skills and abilities. And while you are playing up your skills and abilities, try to do it somewhat modestly. Sound hard? It is, but like anything else, interviewing is something that you get better at the more you do it.

Don't be afraid to speak up during an interview. This is the time to say you are a good student or that you won an important science or writing prize. Point out how your extra-curricular activities might have helped prepare you for this job. If, for example, you are applying for work in a child-care center, comment that you have baby-sat for children of all ages or that your church group has entertained orphans for five Christmases and that you have been in charge of leading the songfest. If the work you are applying for is largely secretarial, mention your good grades in English. Before you go into an interview, you should review your experiences to see how they might fit in with this job you hope to get.

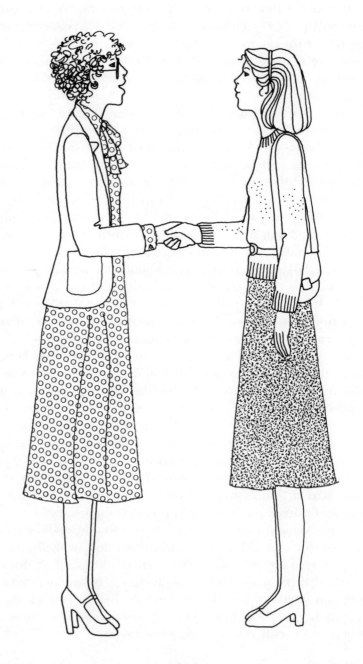

166

Another way to impress a prospective employer is to note that the job he is offering would provide you with an opportunity to explore an area in which you might want to work in the future. You might tell a hospital director, for example, that you hope to get a part-time laboratory job because you think you want to be a doctor someday, and you're sure the experience of working in a hospital will prove invaluable.

You do indeed have to walk a fine line between bragging and modesty in a job interview, but most important is that you sell yourself to a prospective employer. If necessary, role-play an interview with a friend, or better yet, with a guidance counselor at school or some other adult who can advise you.

Finally, avoid appearing cocky or flirtatious. You may be wowing all the boys at school with your charms, but this won't work on an interview. Be polite and friendly but somewhat reserved—*especially* if you are interviewing with a family friend. If you go to work for a family friend, he or she will want to know that you won't take advantage of the situation—and maintaining a reserved attitude during the interview is one way of showing this.

Do a little homework before you go on the interview and, if possible, mention what you have learned. You need to know something about the company and the job—things such as how long the company has been in business, what they produce or what service they provide, what their reputation is, how many people work for them.

Ask specific questions about the job. It shows you are interested, and it shows that you have a good sense of business. Just be sure to ask questions directly related to the nature of the work and not such things as how long a lunch hour you will be allowed or whether you can leave early on Friday afternoons. And keep personal things out of the interview—the person talking to you doesn't care whether your boyfriend works in a competing company or is captain of the basketball team.

Talking Money

Unfortunately, teens are pretty much at the mercy of the marketplace when salary comes up. If you have previous job experience or have earned more than is being offered on this job, however, you may have some ammunition for negotiating a better salary than the initial offer. When salary is discussed, you might say, "Well, I earned $20 more a week last summer, and I also have the dictaphone experience that you said was optional, so I feel that might make me worth a little more money."

Mostly, though, you take what is offered and keep dreaming about the day when you will have the education and experience to command an outstanding salary.

If the job has been offered and you have accepted it, do be sure that you understand what you will be paid and when you are to start work before you leave the interview. If you have not been offered a job, ask if you can call next week to see whether or not a decision has been made.

Following Up on an Interview

If a job is left open, it is usually up to you to find out when it is filled. This also shows enthusiasm—a very necessary ingredient of job hunting—and emphasizes that you are eager to get the job, if possible.

Call back in a week or so to ask whether or not a decision has been made. Then call back in another week to ask the same thing. If you do this politely, most persons will not mind.

Also, when someone has taken the time to interview you for a job, write a brief thank-you note expressing again your interest in the job and noting that you appreciated the time spent talking with you.

If possible, this note and any other business correspondence should be typed. Business communications books show the proper format for a business letter—check one out of the school library and read the chapters that apply to job hunting.

Job hunting is hard work, but it's also fun. And it's experience that you will use throughout your life. The more you interview, the more letters you write and phone calls you make, the better at it you will become—and the more you will increase your chances of being at ease on your next important interview. Happy job hunting!

15

THE YOUNG MEN
IN YOUR LIFE

⋙ At some point in your teen years, you will undoubtedly become interested in boys—and that's probably when you will think your life is suddenly very complicated and more than a little strange. Dating is an entirely new adventure, and one that gets better with a little practice.

Getting Along with Boys

Whatever growing pains you are suffering, it's important to remember that boys have their own set of worries and problems. For one thing, they are suddenly surrounded by girls who are starting to look like women, and suddenly they are getting feelings about those girls that they are not sure how to handle. Partly they are sexual and emotional feelings, and partly they are just feelings about how to deal with girls socially, since this is obviously what is now called for. Then, too, everyone matures at a different rate. Your best friend may have discovered the charms of boys a year before you did, and the same thing happens to boys. You may get interested in a boy who just isn't quite ready to be interested in you. When this happens, you had better seek other companionship and wait for him to grow up a little more.

Even the boys who are interested in girls are usually scared to death. But boys have been brought up to feel that they are not supposed to act scared, and they *are* supposed to take the lead in dealing with girls. This is why you will have to put up with strange behavior sometimes—teasing, or a boy who engages you in a long conversation as if he's going to ask you out but obviously can't muster up the courage to do so, or one perfectly pleasant date that is not followed by a second date of any kind.

Once you realize that boys basically are even less sure of themselves than girls are, they become somewhat easier to deal with. And here are a few more hints: Don't chase boys. Don't expect great masculine things from them. Do treat them like friends. Do be and act as if you are sincerely interested in them. The best way to practice for a romantic relationship with a boy is to be some boy's good friend for a while. Your friend may never turn into a romance (then again, he might), but you will be able to develop some insight into what goes on in his mind.

What do boys generally expect from girls? Our talks with teenage boys showed that they mostly like "natural" girls— the ones who make them feel at ease and do not flirt with them to the point of embarrassment. Most boys opt for little makeup and girls who dress right for the occasion, whatever it is. Femme fatale and chorus line looks are especially frightening to boys. They may not have any idea how much you spend on clothes, or whether or not your clothes are home-sewn or come from the fanciest boutique in town, but they do know whether or not you are dressed for an occasion.

Giving Your First Party

A sure sign that you are developing an interest in boys is the urge to give a party to which you think about inviting girls *and* boys.

First parties, too, are often scary, but they need not be if you have an idea of what is expected of you as the party-giver.

First of all, keep in mind why you are giving a party: you want to treat your friends, girls and boys alike, to an enjoyable event. As hostess, you will want to be gracious to everyone and make everyone feel as comfortable as possible in your home.

Once you've drawn up a guest list, it's time to issue invitations. You can send written ones (make sure to include time, place, occasion if any, and your name and telephone number), or you can simply ask people informally when you see them. Asking people informally is probably the best way—just be sure you ask everyone you intend to. When you ask someone, be direct but make the person feel that you really want him or her to come. This is not the time for a sarcastic crack such as, "If you aren't nice to me, I won't invite you to my house Saturday night with the rest of the kids." How can anyone respond to that? Instead, you might say, "By the way, Jack, I'm having a bunch of people over Friday after the game. I hope you can come. You can? Great. Here, let me write my address for you and give you some simple directions. Gee, I'm glad you'll be there. See you then."

Once you've gotten your party in the works by extending invitations, you'll need to prepare for your guests. Fortunately, the ingredients that guarantee success at a teen party are simple: lots of good food, popular music, casual dress, and maybe some games or dancing.

The food you serve depends upon the occasion. Plan to have a wide selection of soft drinks on hand. You can have bowls of potato chips and nuts sitting around, but you should also plan to bring on something a little heartier at some point during the evening. This can be simple—hot dogs or hamburgers and potato salad are always hits, for example.

As your guests arrive, have music playing in the background —not so loud they can't talk, but not so softly that everyone will feel like listening instead of dancing.

Greet each person at the door; take your guest's coat or tell the guest where to put it; and when the guest rejoins the party, introduce him or her to someone. If possible, introduce a guest to a small group that is easy to break into conversationally. Try to use first and last names and to make the introduction personal, but if the group is large, a quick exchange of first names may have to do.

Be prepared with some planned activity, but don't force it on your guests. Putting on dance music and asking one couple to start dancing should be enough to get dancing off the ground if your guests are interested. Have some games around that your guests can naturally gravitate toward if they are so inclined. If you want to play a game as a group, suggest it and show enthusiasm for it, but don't press if the rest of the crowd doesn't show much interest.

Most teens have curfews of some sort, so the party will probably end of its own accord. If the party goes on really late, the appearance of your parents or a few subtle acts of cleaning up on your part (take away the potato-chip dish and *don't* bring it back refilled) should give your guests the message that the evening can end anytime.

A party is a good way to mix all sorts of people and to introduce some of your friends to other friends they have not met. It is also the perfect way to show interest in a boy. Ask him to the party and make a point of talking with him sometime during the evening. A party is also a good way to get a group of friends together when you don't have a date—no one will think anything one way or another about whether you have a date.

Meeting Boys

There are lots of ways to meet boys, but one thing is certain: you can't meet them by staying at home. The best way is the most obvious: go where they are. This includes parties, school activities, sports events, Y-group activities, clubs, and hobby or interest groups. In fact, hobby or interest groups are among the best ways to meet boys. You have gone somewhere to follow up on an interest. Boys like girls who have strong interests, and meeting a boy through an interest group automatically means you have something to talk about.

Meeting a boy without benefit of a formal introduction is easy. All you have to do is smile. Don't make a cute remark— it just sounds dumb—but do be prepared to talk when a boy walks over and says something to you (or you can walk over to him). Ask him why he is attending the meeting, lecture, museum, whatever. Then, when the first awkward silence arrives, ask him about another interest or about sports or even where he goes to school. Questions that sound slightly boring ("How do you like all this snow we're getting?") may actually be an immense relief to the boy who's frantically trying to think of what to say next.

Don't fill every minute with talk, though. It's surprising what a person will say to you when you let a conversation lapse. In fact, that's often the very moment when a boy will say, "How would you like to go to a movie Saturday night?"

When a Boy Calls on the Phone

More often than not, a boy won't ask you out the first time you meet him. He may choose instead to call you on the phone. Keep in mind that even this is a big move for a teenage boy. Boys don't spend hours on the phone the way teenage girls often do.

When you pick up the phone, and a boy is on the other end, be prepared to help him out a little. Start by making him feel that you are happy to hear from him. Even go so far as to start a conversation. You could say, "Oh, John, how are you? Did you finish working on your car? I saw that you were hard at work when I was walking home today."

Lulls in a telephone conversation can be worse than long lulls in face-to-face conversation. You may have to bring up still another topic. If the boy never seems to pick up the lead and he doesn't ask you out as you expect or hope, don't drag out the conversation. Generally, the person who does the calling is the one to sign off, but some boys don't know this. When the conversation is going nowhere or has apparently come to an end (maybe he only did want to ask you about your math assignment), sign off sweetly and politely.

If you met a boy somewhere but don't remember him and he calls, admit that you don't remember him. He'll give you some information to jog your memory, and you can decide whether or not you want to go out with him if he asks you.

When You Call a Boy on the Phone

It's true that women have equal rights these days, especially where men are concerned, but phone calls from girls may not be a feminist issue to a teenage boy. Try not to call boys unless you have a legitimate reason to do so. Just calling to chat is liable to scare a boy so much that he will never call you. Legitimate reasons to call include such things as an inquiry about his health if he has been ill, a school question, an invitation to a girl-asks-boy event, a word of congratulations or consolation if something good or bad has happened to him.

Keep phone calls to boys brief and to the point. If he brings up a new conversation, by all means talk with him, but don't plan to go on for hours or even for very many minutes.

Accepting a Date

There will come a day when a phone call or a meeting will lead to that all-important invitation—your first real date. Stay calm when it happens. Act interested. Get the details of the date—where and when, what you need to wear or bring, etc. Thank the boy for asking you and tell him that you're looking forward to seeing him.

Declining a Date

You must decline a date when you have already made plans, and you may want to decline a date if you don't want to go out with a particular person. There are ways to do each.

If you want to go out with the boy sometime, tell him you are sorry that you already have plans and say that you hope he will call again. If you have a chance, repeat this or thank him again for asking you out. If he asks if you would like to go to a movie on Friday, and you can't, you might say, "But how about next Friday?" or "Would you like to come over to study on Tuesday?"

If someone you do not want to go out with asks you out, a slightly different tactic is called for. Say no graciously, but don't give a reason. If the boy doesn't get the message after you have turned him down this way several times, you might say that you are already seeing someone or that you are too busy to go out for a while.

Your First Date—and Other Dates

No matter how nervous you are, try to act relaxed. Remember that the boy is probably more nervous than you are, and he certainly feels more of the responsibility for making this evening go well.

Be ready when your date picks you up. Introduce him to your parents if they are home and chat with them for a minute or two. You can be the one to suggest leaving.

Once you are out with your date, be on your best behavior. Act as if you've done this a few times before. Be polite to people who wait on you. Be fairly quiet, or at least don't be rowdy. Always respect property wherever your date has taken you.

Be gracious to your date, too. Thank him for any courtesies he shows you, such as opening a door or helping you into your coat. Compliment him, either personally or for some part of the evening. If you go to a hamburger hangout after a movie, for example, comment on how good the food tastes. Don't pan a movie he has taken you to unless he starts the conversation. Above all, if you know you want to see him again, thank him warmly for the evening.

During the date, let your companion be a gentleman if he is so inclined. If you have strong feminist feelings, and you really wish he wouldn't make you sit in the car while he comes around to open the door, you can drop this into a conversation later. First time out, though, let him lead and see what courtesies he is inclined to show you. On the other hand, don't press a boy to show you more courtesy than he thinks necessary. One boy said, "I know I'm supposed to get into taxis first, but it always seems so awkward that I just open the door and stand there until my date gets in." If a boy doesn't present quite the array of manners you like, you can either ignore this and hope to polish him up later when you know him better or you can find someone else. Nagging or otherwise expressing your discontent won't work.

Manners on Dates

There are a few courtesies that boys show to girls and women, and you should be prepared for these on a date. First, there is the question of who goes first. In a restaurant, you follow the hostess or maître d'hôtel, if there is one. If you seat yourselves, you follow your date to your table. In cabs and buses, technically your date gets in and out first, but in practice boys and men often stand back and let a girl or woman go first. Girls usually go through doors ahead of boys.

It's not good manners to ask a boy to carry things that belong to you in his pockets. You shouldn't even expect him to carry your books if you are both weighed down with them, but if he is empty-handed, he should offer—or you could ask him—to help you with your packages. Then, if you see him carrying a lot of stuff, you might offer to help him. Manners really have more to do with people being courteous to each other than with a stuffy set of rules that must be followed to a T.

Breaking a date is rude. Once you have accepted an invitation to go somewhere, you should back out only if you are ill or if there is illness in your family, if your family has something planned that you didn't know about when you accepted and must attend, if out-of-town guests show up unexpectedly, or if you have to go out of town.

Your First Kiss, Etc.

At some point, most likely during your teen years, *it* will happen. You will kiss or be kissed for the first time. There really are not any specific hints or guidelines that anyone can give you for this occasion, except to promise that you will know what to do when it happens. Some things in life just work themselves out naturally, and kissing is one of those things.

Once you have kissed a few boys a few times, you will have another kind of problem—what kind of physical relationship you want with a boy or boys you are dating. Whether or not you are ready for a serious relationship with a boy is something you will have to devote a lot of thought to, will have to work out yourself. You do have help in this area. There are lots of books on the subject, a school counselor may be willing to talk with you, or your mother may not be too shy to discuss sex with you. You could also turn to an older sister or a friend's older sister, if you need someone to talk with. Then, too, you will have lots of opportunities to listen to your friends, but they may not be your best resource. Teenage boys are notorious for talking after the event about their sexual activity, but teenage girls also often overestimate to their friends how comfortable they are when they become heavily involved physically with a boy. You may want to keep this in mind when a friend is encouraging you to try something you aren't comfortable with. In the end, the decision about what kind of physical relationship you will have with a boy is yours. You must do what you are comfortable with—and no more.

Boys Have Feelings, Too

The fact that boys and men often show their emotions less than women do does not mean that they can't be hurt. Be careful of a boy's feelings. Show him the same tact and friendship that you would direct to a girlfriend.

Don't flirt with other boys when you are out with someone, and don't talk about other boys you have dated. Also, don't lead a man on. You aren't more popular because lots of boys have asked you to go steady or told you they love you; you're simply a scalp-hunter. You can tell when a boy is starting to care more about you than you care about him, and this is the time to cool things off gently.

Be Careful of Yourself

It is important to know how to take care of yourself on a date. Years ago, boys and girls did not date. A boy could only call on a girl at her parents' home, and when they became engaged he might be allowed to take her out for a walk alone. Today, socializing between boys and girls is much less formal, and you may even go out with a boy you've met somewhere on your own before you've been formally introduced by a mutual friend. This is okay, but it does call for a little care and common sense.

Be a little leery when going out for the first time with someone you don't know well. Plan an activity in a public place— a movie or a snack in a school hangout. On your first date with a boy you don't know well, it is best not to accept an invitation to his house unless you know it is for a party, or even to a party where you don't know anyone else. If possible, suggest that you double date with your friends.

Whether you are out with someone you don't know well or an old family friend, admit to having a curfew. Most teens do, especially when they start dating. Tell your date early in the evening what time you have to be home so it doesn't sound as if you made up the curfew to cut the date short.

If your date suggests going somewhere that you don't like— a place where the kids drink, for example—just tell him you would rather go somewhere else. You never have to go along with a date or the crowd when you know it would be better not to.

If your date is a wild driver, comment, but try to do it tactfully. Your life, however, is at stake, and you have every right to say something about driving—especially about driving and drinking.

By the time you are an older teen, you may be going out with boys who are legally old enough to drink even though you aren't. Mostly, the laws of your state should help you handle this situation. You may not be allowed to go into bars, or you won't be allowed to order alcoholic beverages even if you can go into a bar. The temptation to drink or to feel grown-up because your date is drinking is a big one, but it is also dangerous. Just because the law says someone is old enough to drink does not mean that person is emotionally ready to do so, and it almost certainly never means that a teenage boy has had enough experience to drink and then drive you home. If the drinking has become a problem, offer to drive home, call a cab, or share a ride with some friends. Drinking and driving never mix, and you have every reason to refuse to get into a car with someone who has been drinking.

Finally, it is reasonable—even in these days of women's liberation—to expect a boy to pick you up and return you home safely at the end of a date. There may be informal occasions when you will be willing to meet your date somewhere, but you should still expect to be taken home after dark. It's not a matter of courtesy; it's a matter of safety.

Blind Dates

Most teens with any dating experience quickly develop feelings about blind dates. Either you are willing to take the risk or you are not. Blind dates can be fun, and you should at least try one or two before you rule them out forever. The biggest mistake most people make about blind dates is expecting too much. If you haven't found Prince Charming on your own, why expect him to show up on a blind date? Keep this in mind, and don't raise your expectations for a blind date. Do, however, give the boy a chance before you decide he's a dud.

Try to talk to a blind date on the phone before you accept an invitation. If you decide, based on what you hear, that you really won't get along, then tell him that. Gently say that you don't think you have much in common and maybe it would be better not to see each other on a date.

If you think there is the slightest possibility that you will get along (and remember how hard it is to convey personality over the phone), then make a date. Don't, however, let much time elapse between your acceptance and the actual date. This only creates tension and too-high expectations—the bane of blind dates. And when you go out with the boy, relax and have fun. It's only one evening out of your life.

Double Dates

Either you or the boy you are going out with may suggest that you double with another couple. Couples nowadays sometimes even ask a single friend to join them. Go out of your way to be pleasant to people you double with. If you really dislike them, you can possibly discuss this with your date later, but don't ruin everyone's evening by not acting graciously.

Going Dutch

Who pays for what on a date depends upon custom in your circle of friends, how long you have dated the boy (couples who go out a lot together are more likely to share expenses), and how you both feel about going Dutch. Regardless of who pays most of the time, on special occasions—such as when he asks you to a school dance or you ask him to a dance or other special function—the person who does the asking should pay for the tickets and major expenses connected with the evening.

If you do go Dutch, there are several ways to do it. You could give your date some money at the beginning of the evening, and he could settle with you at the end. You could pay as you go along. Or you could switch off, letting one person pay for the movie one week and the other person pay the following week, or by letting one person pay for the movie and the other pay for the after-movie snack.

If money is a real problem for someone you are dating, you should tactfully do whatever you can to help him. Don't suggest expensive dates you know a boy can't afford. Ask him over to study or play records with you. Look for free activities you can enjoy together. If you really want to do something special, such as go to a symphony or a play, buy the tickets and say that they were given to you. You could even arrange to be given a special dinner out by your parents. Don't overuse this tactic, though, or it will soon become obvious that you are supporting this relationship in a way that the boy cannot afford to.

Dressing for Dates

Boys especially appreciate girls who dress appropriately for dates. Asking what you will be doing should provide you with a clue about what to wear. If you aren't sure what to wear, check with other girls to see what they are wearing. Most dates are either casual, sports-oriented, dressy-informal, or formal. Casual dates call for jeans or pants or possibly a skirt and a nice shirt or sweater. For sports dates, wear whatever is called for—tennis whites for a tennis date, a loose skirt or pants for a bowling date, ski clothes for skiing, casual clothes for roller or ice skating, and very warm clothes for any outdoor winter sports. It's no fun for you or the boy if you dress inappropriately for outside activity.

A dressy-informal date can be dinner out, dinner at the home of your date, or even a school dance. You may wear anything from a skirt and sweater or dressy separates to a nice dress. Each school generally has its own fashions for an informal dance, and you will want to wear whatever is acceptable at your school. A formal dance calls for an evening dress.

Proms and Dances

As exciting as your first boy-girl party or your first date is, few things rival your first invitation to a prom or formal dance. Even the anticipation is fun, and there is truly a lot to do to get ready. First, determine what dress will be appropriate, for you will want to wear pretty much what everyone else is wearing. You will want to wear an evening dress, but the styles that teens consider evening dress vary from year to year and from community to community. Sometimes a black velvet evening skirt and dressy silk blouse is what you need; in the summer or spring floor-length cotton dresses may be the order of the evening; at other times you will want a stunning, fancy evening dress. Before you choose something, check with other girls who are attending to see what their dresses will be like.

When shopping for a prom or dance dress, you will find a variety of gowns designed especially for teens. Still, you may be tempted to wear something too sophisticated for you. Try to avoid this temptation, for your first dance is a time to look stunning, radiant, innocent—*and* your age. Choose a white or pastel dress, and do not succumb to black. No matter how grown-up you feel wearing it in the dressing room, it won't make it on the dance floor for your school prom. If you buy a very dressy fabric such as satin or silk, be sure that the style is young enough for you. Chiffon dresses rarely look young enough for teenagers to carry off, but you may find a dress that is the exception.

Once you have gotten your dress, the next step is to find the right accessories. You will need shoes, gloves, an evening purse, and a wrap that looks good with your dress.

Your shoes can be a dressy silver, gold, or other-colored sandal, or you may want to buy pumps and have them dyed to match.

Traditionally, long, over-the-elbow gloves are worn with an evening dress, but don't fall into the trap of thinking you must wear gloves this length. If your dress looks better with shorter—say, wrist-length—gloves, then this is what you should wear.

Evening purses are small, and may be either clutch or shoulder strap. They are usually made of a dressy fabric such as satin, faille, brocade, silk, or beads, but a pretty mock or real suede or leather purse in a dressy style could work well.

A coat is usually your biggest problem. Lucky you if the prom is at a time of year when the weather is warm enough so you only need a pretty, dressy shawl. For blustery winter evening dances, you have to find something else to wear. If you can make your dressy winter coat work, do so. If you can afford a matching or fancy evening coat, that's also a possibility. About the only thing that does not work on a teen is a fancy fur coat. Your mother's mink stole, jacket, or coat will only look silly and slightly ostentatious, so resist the urge to borrow it. If you own a nice modest fur coat, by all means wear that.

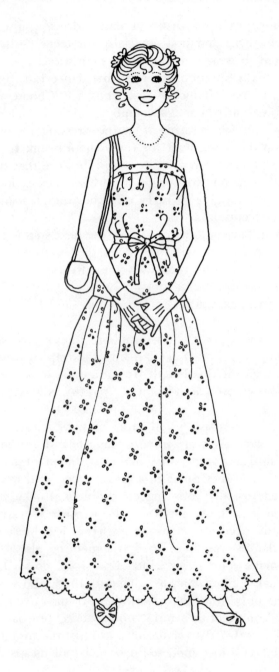

In addition to getting yourself ready for the prom, make sure that your date knows what he is expected to wear. If he doesn't ask, you may want to hint that flowers are called for, but never suggest what kind of flowers you would like. The boy is supposed to bring what he can afford.

If you really think your date won't know that flowers are expected, you could, as an emergency measure, order a flower to wear in your hair or on your dress. It should not be a corsage, but, rather, should look as if it were needed to complete your "look." Flowers are worn stem down, the way they grow. Use a concealed safety pin rather than a corsage pin to attach the flowers with slightly more security.

The Big Night

When your date calls for you, he will undoubtedly tell you how lovely you look—and you should respond by telling him how handsome he looks.

You *will* feel different—like a princess, like an elegant model, or maybe even like an old-fashioned belle—dressed up so beautifully. By all means, walk a little more serenely and royally to secretly play out your role if you like. You should not, however, be so stiff and formal that neither you nor your date can relax and have fun. Remember that your date probably feels slightly awkward dressed in his evening clothes (boys don't fantasize about their first evening suit the way girls do about their first evening dress), so it is up to you to set an easy tone for the evening. Do use your best manners and walk in a way that shows off you and your lovely dress, but stop short of overdoing it.

Arriving at a Dance

When you arrive at the dance, check your coat and refresh your makeup in the ladies' room. If the weather is cold, and you are wearing a coat, carry your flowers in their box to the dance and put them on after you get there. You can check your gloves or keep them, but if you keep them with you plan to wear them. You can wear gloves when dancing or meeting people, but remove them completely when eating.

Rejoin your date and go through the receiving line together, if there is one. Receiving lines sound formidable until you have gone through one and found out just how easy they are. Simply step up to the beginning of the line and say, "Hello, my name is Susanna Farraday." The person in the line will say hello and mention his name in return and may make a comment or ask a brief question before he or she passes you on to the next person in the line. If you know someone in the receiving line, simply greet him naturally. Don't stop for a prolonged conversation in a receiving line; the idea is to move through it fairly quickly.

Getting Rid of a Bore

Sometimes you will find yourself talking too long with someone who does not particularly interest you. There are several polite ways to get rid of him. Excuse yourself and go to the ladies' room. When you return, join another group. Or you can get refreshments and work your way, with this person, into a group that you can mingle with. If worse comes to worse, and you feel you have spent enough time with him, simply say, "Excuse me, I have to talk to someone," and walk over to a group of friends.

Dancing Cheek to Cheek—or Otherwise

The purpose of a dance is *to dance,* so there is little reason for you to be unwilling to do just that. If you cannot dance when you get invited to one, take lessons or ask a friend to show you the latest steps before the dance. You can even learn the most popular dances as you go along on the dance floor. Don't worry about your skills as a dancer. Most people are only average dancers, anyway.

There are a few things to watch when you are dancing:

• Don't dance in a death grip with your partner. Save any serious affection you want to show each other for a quiet time alone. Dancing in the throes of passion looks silly and makes others feel ill at ease.

• Don't hum while you dance.

• Don't sing while you dance.

• Don't gesture or talk to your friends while you dance.

• Keep a pleasant expression on your face while dancing, even if the boy is walking all over your feet.

• Let the boy lead. Someone has to, and traditionally this has been his role.

Don't spend all night dancing with your date. Dances and parties are social occasions, and you should be in a festive enough mood to want to mingle with everyone there. Your date will probably have to excuse himself anyway to dance with the chaperones and the hostess before the dance ends, and this is a good time to accept dances from other boys. Actually, you can accept dances from other boys at any time—even if they cut in on you when you are dancing with your date. When you have finished a dance with someone, he will probably thank you. Thank him in return or simply smile graciously.

The Weekend Visit

You may be asked to a dance or prom at a boy's school or in his hometown, if he lives in a community other than yours. Often these invitations are for the whole weekend. Perhaps most thrilling of all is to be asked to your first college weekend.

When a boy calls to ask you for a weekend visit, and you plan to go, get all the details. You need to know how to get there, the length of your stay, the events you will attend, the clothes you will need, and where you will stay. With these facts in hand, carefully plot out everything you will need for the weekend. Since you will be operating, more or less, on

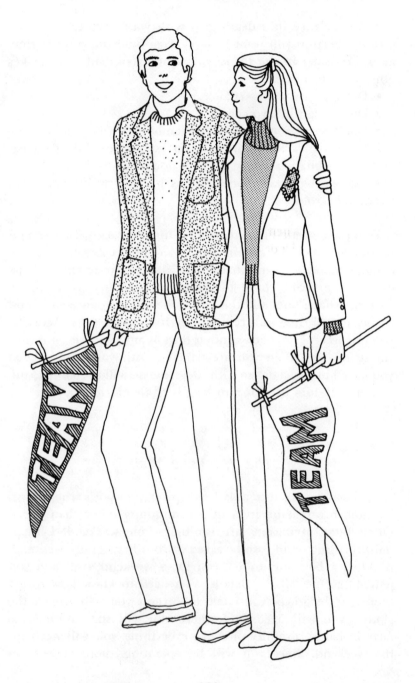

strange terrain, take everything you will need. Don't count on borrowing some other girl's hair blower or electric rollers, and especially don't count on borrowing any accessories to go with your evening dress or clothes.

If the boy does not arrange a ride for you, you must arrange your own transportation; your date will undoubtedly tell you what is available and how to get there, however.

On a college or prep school weekend, you usually pay for your transportation, any meals you eat alone, your miscellaneous expenses, and you should offer to pay for your room. Your date may or may not have already paid for your room.

Weekend dates are special occasions not only to girls but also to boys. Once you have accepted an invitation, you owe it to your date to be gracious to him and his friends *all* weekend. Displays of temper, expressions of disappointment over your living quarters, dismay because your date cannot be with you every single minute are all ungracious and will result in your getting fewer invitations to exciting college weekends.

Sometimes you will want to ask a boy to attend a special function or dance at your school. If possible, and if he has to travel any distance, ask him for the entire weekend. When this happens, you shoulder pretty much the same responsibilities that he shouldered for you: finding him a room and paying for any major entertainment over the weekend. Be sure he knows what clothes are required for the events planned.

Weekend Visits to His Home

You will occasionally be asked to be a weekend guest at a boy's home, particularly if he lives any distance from you. He may extend the invitation informally, but his mother will also write a brief note inviting you, too. You should reply to her note in writing.

It goes without saying that you will want to be on your best behavior during this visit. Offer to help his mother with any household tasks you see her doing. Bring appropriate clothes so you can participate in whatever your date or his family are doing at the moment. Join in whatever family activities are planned. If you hate tennis, and his family spends every minute on the courts, then this is what you should do for this weekend. Also, bring along a book and be prepared to spend some time alone. No one wants to have to entertain a house-guest every single minute, and your willingness to amuse yourself alone for a while will only endear you to your host and hostess.

You pay your travel and phone expenses while you are visiting; either your date or his family will pay for anything else.

Most important, treat your relationship with the boy with great care. He is exposing his feelings to you by asking you to meet and spend time with his family. Don't overwork your relationship by acting possessive. And don't get caught in a compromising position. He may just casually drop by your room and you may become involved in an entirely innocent conversation while sitting on the bed, but it probably won't look innocent if his mother walks by. And his mother will most likely think that you instigated her son's visit to your room, that being the way of mothers. So you take full responsibility for not putting yourself in any kind of compromising position that could force his parents to have second thoughts about you.

Finally, leave at the appointed time. You may be encouraged to take a later train or stay over another night, but remember that it's always nice to exit while you are still wanted. Don't change your plans—at least not the first time you visit someone.

And when you return home, write his mother and the boy each a short note thanking them for the weekend. If you feel like it, you could send his mother a small hostess gift.

Correspondence

Romance by mail is a lot of fun, and even boys who are not good correspondents enjoy getting letters. You can even use the mail to show interest in a boy who hasn't yet gotten the hint that you like him. Send him an amusing cartoon or a clipping of an article on a subject that you know interests him. Don't overdo this, though. One message is enough unless he replies and shows a willingness to spark a friendship. Girls who constantly send "cute" cards to boys don't win their friendship; they embarrass them.

And when you are exchanging letters with someone you date, pace your letters according to how often you hear from him. If he waits three weeks or even a month to reply to your letter, don't answer him right away; rather, wait about the same amount of time and then write him. Don't send off daily or even weekly letters unless you are getting the same response.

Make your letters cheerful and amusing. Put funny drawings in the margins or tell a funny story about something that happened to you. Don't overdo the romance by mail with flowery or perfumed paper, and don't write intensely romantic or passionate things in letters. More often than not, sweet nothings look silly. Also, be careful not to write things that have double meanings. If, for example, you attended a dance together at a major downtown hotel, don't write, "I will never forget the night we spent together at the Plaza." There is a chance that someone in his family—or worse, a teasing classmate—will latch on to a letter like this and torture him with it. Stick to light, amusing letters and you will be more assured of getting a response and of having your letters eagerly awaited.

Gifts

If you have been seeing a boy regularly for some time, and a major cause for celebration comes along, you will probably want to buy him a present. Most boys aren't sensitive to such minor events as Valentine's Day, so either don't bother buying him anything or get him something very small that you won't mind not giving him if he doesn't give you something first.

Go light on buying a gift for a boy, anyway. Anything too

expensive or too personal is likely to embarrass him. Records, books, and games make excellent presents. They're fun to receive, and they don't scream, "I love you" too much. Expensive items of clothing or inexpensive ones that say, "I want to take care of you"—this includes socks, robes, and scarves—are better left to later, more serious romances; in fact, they are better left to his mother's gift list.

Gifts aren't something a boy can hide from his family or roommates, and it's a rare boy who appreciates an elaborate show of affection demonstrated by a gift that is too expensive or too personal.

Breaking Up—When You End It

Once you know that a relationship with a boy isn't right, it is time to break it off. As painful as this may sound, it is easier and kinder than prolonging it.

If you have only been dating someone every once in a while, you can sometimes simply say no when you are asked out. After a few refusals, the boy will usually get the hint. Better still, have a talk with him and explain that you are seeing someone else or that you are too busy at school to go out for a while.

Even after you have broken up with someone, always be nice to him when you see him. Say hello and ask how he is. Show as much interest in his life as you can, but don't flirt—he may take that to mean that you have suddenly developed renewed interest in him.

Breaking Up—When He Ends It

There is nothing you can do if a boy you really like decides to break up with you. Often teenage boys are so inexperienced in this department that their way of breaking up is simply to not call a girl they have been seeing again. Keep in mind that this has to do with his immaturity and not with anything you have done.

If he does tell you he wants to break up, be as gracious as possible. To salvage your pride, you might even agree and say that you had been thinking you would like to date around.

Don't ask him why, or ask any other pleading questions. It won't change anything. And you will only feel embarrassed the next time you see him. By letting him down gently, you will give him a chance to think better of you than he might otherwise.

Getting Back in Circulation

If you have been dating someone steadily for a while, you may wonder how you are going to get back into the swing of things. It's easy. Plan to do things with your girlfriends. Pass the word to all your friends that you are looking for someone to go out with. Go to parties. Have a party—and ask that new boy you have been eyeing.

The Art of Getting Along with Boys

Actually, there is no art to getting along with boys. Treat them as people. Be relaxed and casual around them, and for those times when you get nervous about being with them, remember that teenage boys are much more frightened than teenage girls about the socializing that goes on during these years.

16

HOW TO BE
A SOCIAL SUCCESS

◄§ Social success is something you can make happen. It does require some skills, but most of those skills are simply good manners and an appreciation of how to treat others so they will like you and enjoy your company.

Be True to Yourself

You do have to be a little realistic about where you fit in. Many teens spend hours lamenting the fact that they are not members of the "popular" crowd. Some teens seem naturally to gravitate to the cheerleaders and the class leaders, and other teens—the ones you may not have noticed before—ignore that crowd in favor of finding or making their own niches—perhaps in drama, on the debate team, as the best girl athlete. While it is nice to be a member of the "popular" crowd, it may not necessarily be the best group for you—and you may be trying to achieve something that will only make you unhappy even if you manage to achieve it.

Two sisters, only a year apart in high school, once had to

work out their feelings about which crowds they would belong to. One sister, naturally outgoing, had belonging to the popular crowd as her main goal. She wanted to be elected an officer of several class organizations; she wanted to go to lots of parties and participate in many activities. It was important to her to date a boy who was a class leader. The other sister, who showed up at the same high school one year later, thought she would follow in her sister's footsteps and run around with the popular crowd. She tried, but she soon discovered that she did not enjoy extracurricular activities. In fact, she preferred to earn extra money baby-sitting after school. She did not particularly like big parties or dances, preferring instead to ask a few friends over to hear records and talk about the books they had been reading. She thought the boys who were class leaders were not nearly as interesting as her old playmate down the block, who was building a complicated entry for the state Science Fair. In fact, the only reason she could think of to strive for membership in the popular group was that it had been her older sister's goal. After about a year of trying, she decided it wasn't worth the effort. She had found her own niche, her own interests, and most important, her own friends who made her feel happy and whom she could feel happy about. Sounds simple enough, doesn't it? Yet entire high school "careers" have been ruined because a person constantly thought of social success only in terms of belonging to the "in" crowd. Such people usually emerge from high school with only a few real friends, and with even fewer real interests.

The best thing to remember, then, about social success is to be true to yourself. If you are totally enamored of the popular crowd and nothing much else outside their activities and parties appeals to you, you probably should run with that group. If you are a late bloomer, or are shy, then set your sights on a group with which you can feel comfortable. If you are more interested in books and the debate team, or in science, then let your clique be the people you meet when following up on these interests.

Being a Good Friend

Although boys may appear to be the most important thing
in your life much of the time, the support and friendship of
other girls should never be underestimated. Girls are around
to go to the movies with on those Saturday nights when you
don't have a date. Girls are the people who share many of your
experiences and to whom you can tell your deepest secrets.
Girls are, in short, your best support system. And having good
friends takes a little effort. You have to give in order to get.

The best way to be a good friend to someone is to show a
genuine interest in her. You need to truly care what happens

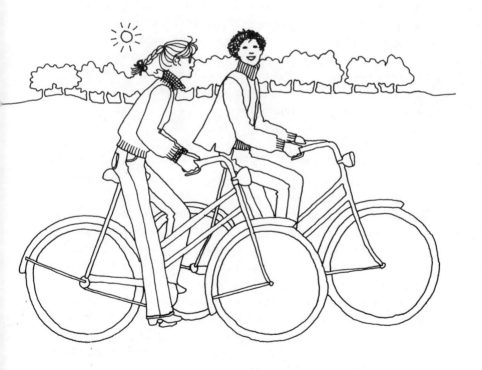

to a friend. If a friend gets a bad report card, show sympathy and even offer to help her study if you can. If a friend has bought a new outfit but isn't sure how she looks in it, offer compliments and support. If a friend is feeling down about a family problem or a boy, be a good listener if she wants to talk about it. Even if a friend's problem is not the same as yours, imagine how you would feel in her situation, and you will find it is easier to respond sympathetically.

Friendship also requires honesty, although even honesty has its limits. A friend wearing a new outfit she has already bought, for example, only wants to hear how good it looks on her. On the other hand, if you are shopping with a friend and she tries on something that you think is unflattering to her, suggest that she looks better in another style or color.

The times when a friend is feeling down are definitely not the times to point out major personality flaws. In fact, the only time you should point out things about someone else's personality is when you find these things interfering with your friendship—and the utmost tact is called for even then. Honesty does demand, however, that you tell a friend when she is doing something that truly offends you.

If a friend has hurt your feelings or offended you, your first reaction might be to pull away, to act cold, or to do something that will hurt or offend her in return. It is not the honest or the sympathetic thing to do, though. Muster up your courage and tell your friend what you would like her to stop doing. She may be talking too much about a boy you just broke up with and would like not to hear about for a while. She may be talking too much about a party that she has been invited to and you haven't. In cases like these, the easiest thing to do is clear the air and discuss what is bothering you.

Two teens we know were best friends since they had been nine; then one of them moved to the other side of town and began to go to another high school. For a while they talked on the phone, and the teen who could drive visited her childhood friend several times. The other teen, who was still too young to drive, felt awkward about maintaining the friendship. She couldn't drive to see her friend, and she didn't think telephone conversations were enough to keep a friendship going—and they were exactly what her friend seemed to be relying on more and more. As a result, she began to let the friendship slip, to avoid calling. Her friend, hurt by these gestures, at least had the common sense to ask what was wrong. And when both girls discussed the difficulties in maintaining a friendship at such a distance, as well as the separate courses their social lives were taking at their different high schools, they soon found themselves feeling closer and wanting to renew their friendship and make sure it stayed intact. They worked out a regular "date" once a month to spend the night with each other and catch up on their lives. Ten years later, both friends are married and have children, but they still meet once a year for a catch-up weekend even though they now live three hundred miles apart. As you can see, friendship takes a little work, but it is worth it.

There are some actions that strain even the best of relationships. Just consider these:

Defensiveness. It's easy when you're new at socializing to be worried about how you are doing. And the natural reaction is one of defensiveness. You may not, for example, take teasing very well. Relax. If someone is really your friend, she will like you no matter what you do. And that means that there is no reason for you to be defensive.

Borrowing. It may not sound as if it belongs on this list, but a lot of teenage friendships have been ruined by this one simple act. Don't borrow and don't lend, if you can avoid it. That way, one entire area of possible hurt feelings will be ruled out. You won't risk being upset if a friend ruins your best outfit or fails to return it.

Easily Hurt Feelings. When you are just beginning to learn how to maneuver socially, it is easy to suffer imagined and real hurts. And the teen years are a time when a lot of things hurt more than they did when you were a child or they will when you are older. So just take it easy. Don't judge your friend's actions too quickly. Give a friend the benefit of the doubt or discuss a problem *before* you end a friendship. Be aware, too, that this is a touchy time for you.

Sarcasm. This seems, in some teen circles, to be the major form of communication. While there is nothing inherently wrong with using sarcasm with your friends, sooner or later it gets out of hand and someone gets hurt. So even if you are a master of sarcasm, lay off once in a while and stop to think how something will feel to someone else.

Gossip. Everyone does it—and there's no use pretending it isn't fun. But gossip hurts other people, and can be particularly harmful when it is false, as is often the case. If you can't avoid it altogether, you should put some limits on it. Try to limit gossip to one or two close friends you truly trust. And never repeat gossip that is truly malicious. This includes personal facts about someone's family life, financial situation, or sexual or love life. If you hear a rumor that someone you know (even vaguely) is pregnant, for example, or that an acquaintance is about to drop out of school because her family needs the money she will earn working, let someone else pass this on. Try to imagine how the other person would feel, and don't you be the carrier of such news.

Finally, when friendships are strained—when you have gone ahead and done some of the things you were just told not to do—admit that you have done something wrong. Apologize when necessary—and even when it isn't absolutely necessary, if it will save a friendship. Overlook a friend's flaws if they don't get in your way too much. No one's perfect, and that includes you.

Getting Along with Your Teachers

Since you spend a large amount of each week in classrooms, you need to know how to get along with your teachers. The most important thing to remember about teachers is that they are people, too. They have interests and activities outside of school, and they also have private lives. The first topic they are quite willing to discuss with you; the second topic is really none of your business. When you meet a teacher socially, don't just talk shop. Ask about movies, books, television shows, or summer travel plans. And no matter how curious you are about your teacher's life, never ask personal questions.

Treat teachers with the same respect you show your friends' parents. Stand to greet them socially (you usually remain seated in classrooms), and call them Mr., Miss (or Ms.), or Mrs. Jones, or whatever their last names are. If you and a teacher leave a room together, let the teacher walk out first as you would with any other adult. In short, show them the courtesy they deserve.

Getting Along with Parents

Into this category fall not only your own parents but also those of your friends. The teenage years can be particularly difficult ones. You are chomping at the bit to get as much freedom as possible, and your parents, believe it or not, are a little frightened about letting you have too many adult responsibilities all of a sudden. Sometimes, family relationships among parents and teens become so tense that it's hard to imagine that you will ever truly like your parents again. (And they undoubtedly have similar feelings about you on occasion.) Yet relations can be considerably eased if everyone involved shows a little understanding. Instead of throwing up your hands in dismay when your parents won't let you do something you want to do, explain quietly and logically *why* you want to do something when you ask permission. If you are about to take a bigger step into the world than you have previously (perhaps by traveling several hundred miles from your home with a group of friends), explain to your parents why you feel you are ready to handle this responsibility. And show them how responsible you are by acting that way as much of the time as possible.

Too often, families fall into patterns of living that seem to ignore the need for good manners. Yet showing courtesy to the people you are closest to is even more important in the long run than showing courtesy to a complete stranger. Make it a habit to impress your family with your good manners. Display good table manners. Don't tie up the telephone or the bathroom for hours on end. Ask in advance when you would like to use a family car for an evening. Most important, pull your weight in doing family chores. Don't let your mother do all the housework, and do help your father with some of his household chores. You should try to do all these things before you are asked, and certainly before you are nagged to do them.

Abide by your parents' rules. Obviously, a little rebellion is part of being a teenager, and you will not always do exactly as your parents want you to do. But if you know your parents feel strongly about your having boys in the house when they are not there, don't do it. To be caught openly defying a rule like that only earns you the mistrust of your parents.

You should try to act according to the rules of your friends' parents as well. If you know that a friend's parents also don't want boys in the house when they aren't home, and you know your friend is planning a party while her parents are out of town for a weekend, remind her of her parents' desires. There are ways to do this without seeming like a goody-goody. And think twice before you go to a party that is unchaperoned. Things can get out of hand with disastrous results.

Certain courtesies are expected to be shown by young adults to older adults. You should stand up when a friend's parents enter the room unless you have already greeted them. You should open doors for parents and other older people and let them walk through first. You should always help an older person with any packages he or she is carrying.

Try to treat a grandparent living in your home or a friend's home with special courtesy. It is sometimes inconvenient to have a much older person living with you, but there are also some wonderful benefits to be gained from friendships with such people.

Breaking into School Groups and Activities

You may have moved to a new school district over the summer, or you may have simply switched schools along with all your peers, but there are a few times when you have to make an effort to break into a group or a club—and there are ways to do this to ensure your success.

First, show an interest in whatever it is that you want to join. You may wait a long time for an invitation to join something, but if you start going to meetings and making your presence felt, you will be asked to participate a lot sooner. There are, of course, some clubs that operate on a principle of exclusivity, and you must wait to be asked to join these. But you may find that you can work your way into a social sorority or other exclusive club by joining other clubs where the people whose special club you hope to join hang out.

Don't, however, befriend people you don't like simply because you want to join a club for the status it offers you. If you don't like the people who belong to the club, no matter how important the club seems to you socially, you probably won't find that membership is worth your efforts.

While you are showing interest, as mentioned earlier, be careful not to take over. At a meeting, for example, make one or two well-thought-out comments or suggestions, but don't monopolize the conversation. Let more established members do most of the talking. Do, on the other hand, volunteer for committee work. It's a chance to show off your organizational skills and become better acquainted with members of the group.

Gradually, people take notice and start to pay more attention to you, and you will soon find yourself with many new friends —as well as a new interest in whatever the club or group is doing.

Inviting Friends Home

As you become closer to someone, you may want to strengthen the friendship by initiating some activities on your own. A comfortable way to get to know someone better is to invite him or her to your home for an after-school snack, to do homework together, to work on some project, or best of all, to just sit around and talk. Check with your mother first to be sure company is convenient. Talk with her about snacks that you can serve.

Explaining Family Problems

During your teen years, when it seems so important to be like your peers, a problem in your family—a retarded sister or brother or an alcoholic parent—may seem like an impossible situation. These things are hard to handle, but they aren't anything you can't learn to cope with.

There is no reason to tell everyone you meet casually about your family problems, but once you have become friends with someone, and you know you would like to invite him or her to your house, you should mention the problem. Explain it matter-of-factly and briefly. Then ask your friend home, if possible.

If someone in the family is too ill for you to bring in outsiders, explain that, too. These situations are nothing to be ashamed of—they are not a reflection of you personally, and if you treat the situation matter-of-factly, your friends will follow your lead.

Overcoming Shyness

Shyness is a funny beast. You can go along for years being the class cut-up or the person who is always picked to introduce school shows, and then suddenly you begin to feel shy about public speaking or meeting others or whatever. Most teens feel shy at one time or another, so you are not alone. And there are some tricks to help you overcome shyness.

First, think about why you have become shy. Most often, it's because you are thrust into new social situations, and you aren't sure how to react. Maybe you are going to parties with boys, and you don't feel totally at ease talking with them. Maybe you are meeting older girls who seem more sophisticated than you, and who leave you feeling tongue-tied. You may not know how to talk to teachers who are suddenly beginning to treat you like an adult. Whatever the cause, you are hit with a case of the "I don't know what to say" blues.

The first step is to learn how to talk to others. And then you must nudge yourself to go out and practice your social skills until they become second nature. Plan in advance what you might possibly discuss with someone. Think of the other person's interests or of something that you find particularly interesting these days and want to discuss. Good subjects to talk about with anyone include movies, television, books, music, your interests, and anything you know the other person is interested in. Boys especially feel comfortable discussing sports, and girls often like to talk about fashions, school activities, and boys—probably in the reverse order.

When you meet a stranger and don't know what to say, a good trick is to think about the other person rather than yourself. One very famous hostess once commented that she finally was able to overcome her shyness when she realized she was talking to someone at a party who was more painfully shy than she was. That made her start thinking that everyone must feel a little awkward in social situations. She began to overcome her shyness by thinking that she was only helping others to be more at ease. Try it and see if it works for you.

If shyness is a real problem, you can make yourself do some little things that may help. Speak to strangers at school, for example. When you get a warm response, as you nearly always will, you will feel better about yourself. Pay other people compliments (sincere ones!)—they are real ice-breakers. Offer to help strangers or old people on the street—you put yourself in the situation of being gracious to someone, and once you have been successful at this you will find it easier to take such risks with people you know.

If you are afraid to speak up in class, talk with a teacher for a few minutes after class. Often the personal exchange will help put you at ease enough to respond in class. You can also try to figure out what questions the teacher may ask and be prepared to answer them. If you know you are going to give the correct answer, it is easier to talk, and you will soon find yourself daring to offer an answer that may not be correct.

As a final resort, you could volunteer for some kind of work that requires you to talk with strangers—a political campaign or a survey, for example. Again, the practice in talking to strangers will bolster your confidence in talking with your peers and teachers.

Carrying on a Conversation

The golden rule of making conversation is to realize that silence is part of the process. No one expects you to talk non-stop. Boys especially are put off by girls who chatter all the time.

The silver rule of making conversation is to learn to be a good listener. Concentrate on what the other person is saying. Ask intelligent questions. Show that you care. Some of the most attractive women in the world are not known for the way they talk, but rather for the way they listen. Think how flattered you are when someone truly listens to you—and then give someone that treatment.

Be funny occasionally. Of course, you can overdo this, too, but serious conversations are for truly old friends. They aren't good at parties.

Don't give a lot of details. No one really wants to hear every question you missed on a test. People especially are not interested in details about illness, personal tragedies, and accidents.

If you realize that a subject is upsetting to someone, back off. People today do tend to discuss controversial issues, such as racism or politics, but if you sense that the person to whom you are talking would rather not talk about these things, be gracious enough to change the subject.

Using Good Manners

You *can* pave the way to social success through the use of good manners. Manners may seem like an outdated notion to you, and indeed they do change from year to year, but they aren't something that most of us are ready to do without yet. Manners basically consist of making others comfortable and doing what is right for you.

There is a way to talk politely on the phone, a way to greet your friends' parents, a way to eat so you don't offend everyone else at the table—there are manners to ease you over almost any situation. And manners will help you feel more at ease.

Cultivate a Pleasant Voice

Although not strictly manners, the cultivation of a pleasant voice is a way to make yourself more attractive to others. It is a very important social asset. Too often, teens resort to loudness or silly talk to get attention when actually, the teen who is poised and who shows this through her speaking voice is more likely to get attention. If possible, take a speech class or practice reading aloud into a tape recorder. Is your voice too loud? Too soft? Too shrill? You can remedy all these things—first, by becoming aware of them, and second, by practicing to change them. Learn to speak slowly and distinctly. Loud, shrill speech is often a signal that you're tense; when you hear yourself talking this way, take a deep breath and start over—or stop talking entirely for a few minutes. When you begin again, your voice will probably be softer and less shrill.

Another part of your voice is what you actually say. Practice the art of talking well without sounding affected or stiff. Do not use foreign words where an English word will do. Don't be afraid to use a good vocabulary, but don't use long words where a shorter word will suffice; this sounds affected, too. Try always to use good grammar. Sometimes teenage slang consists of expressions that are ungrammatical, and while you will undoubtedly want to use the same popular expressions your friends use, be wary of using bad grammar. It might slip out at the wrong time and embarrass you a lot. The same thing goes for swearing. Most teens swear or use some off-color expressions with their friends. In some circles not to do so may brand you as an outsider. Yet most of the time, no one will notice that you aren't using these expressions if you don't make a point of telling anyone why you aren't using them. Try also to avoid such expressions as "I mean" and "you know" when talking; they are boring.

Telephone Manners

Now that you've learned how to speak well, let's talk about telephone manners. You are represented entirely by your voice on the telephone, so it had better be as pleasant as possible. Always answer the phone by saying hello in a pleasant voice. If you are calling a friend's house, identify yourself to whoever answers and ask to speak to your friend: "Hello, Mrs. Smith, this is Jane Jones. Is Sandy there?"

If the person you want to talk with is not at home, leave a message for her or him to call you rather than calling back every ten minutes.

Think about what time it is before you dial. It is not polite to call people during mealtime or late at night. If in doubt, don't call, or check with a friend to see how late you can call.

Table Manners

As your social life becomes more active you will often find yourself in situations where you will be eating with others. Don't let anyone ever tell you that table manners make no difference. You need not follow every minute rule of eating, but no one wants to sit at the same table with a slob. If your parents have not taught you table manners, find a good book at the library and brush up on them. Then practice what you have learned.

Introductions

Throughout your life you will find yourself in situations where you have to introduce one person to another—and there are a few rules to guide you.

When you meet someone yourself for the first time, try to remember his or her name. Repeat it as soon as possible after you hear it the first time, and then use it several times in conversation. That way, you will have the name firmly in mind when you introduce the person to someone else.

Whenever possible, make individual introductions—that is, introduce one person directly to another. If this is not possible, as when you are introducing a friend to a group of friends, then at least mention everyone's first name and say something about the newcomer to the group that will arouse their interest in him. You might say, "Bill, I'd like you to meet some friends from my French club. This is Bob; that's Larry, and Mary, Jenna, Cathy, and Jeremy."

When making more formal, one-to-one introductions, you present one person to another. There are some guidelines for doing this: always present a younger person to an older one (say the older person's name, first, for example, "Mrs. Green, this is Mary Lewis"); always present a guest to a host or hostess; always present someone to a dignitary or a clergyman; always present a student to a teacher; and always introduce men to women. In short, always present someone to a person to whom you wish to show respect or honor.

Among your friends, introductions are much more informal. You simply introduce one person to another, although you may want to stick to the rule of introducing a man to a woman or a boy to a girl.

Boys and men always shake hands when they meet. Women never used to, but young women and girls today have begun to shake hands more often. It's a nice custom, and one you should feel comfortable following if you like it. Generally, a woman or girl is expected to offer her hand to a man or boy, just as an older woman offers her hand when meeting a younger woman.

Writing Letters

At some point, you will have reason to write to someone. And having a regular pen pal or exchanging letters with a good friend is a warm and personal way to communicate.

Stationery comes in all colors, sizes, and shapes these days. You can let your imagination run wild in choosing stationery for writing friends casual letters and notes. For business letters, thank-you notes, and sympathy notes, you need plain white, conservative paper. You can use plain, printed, or engraved writing paper. Envelopes should always match your paper.

Letters—whether casual or official—follow a certain form. Basically, they consist of a greeting, a body, and a closing. You should also date your letters and keep copies of any that are written for business purposes or any that you especially want to copy. Here are suitable greetings:

> Janie—
> Dear Janie,
> Dearest Janie,
> Dear Sir or Ma'am: (for a business letter)
> Dear Mr. Jones: (for a business letter)

Generally, business headings or greetings are followed by a colon, and personal greetings are followed by a comma.

What to Say in a Letter

The body of the letter is the message. It should consist of whatever you want to say. In a business letter you should be brief and to the point. Tell why you are writing and ask for whatever you want: an interview, information, a response to a bill.

There are a few things to think about in writing a personal letter, too. Avoid gloom, if possible. Don't talk at great length about illness, accidents, or personal tragedy. Avoid gossip. Talk lightly about local news, what is happening to people you and the recipient of your letter both know, and what you're doing. Don't give lots of details, but some do spice up a letter. For example, instead of saying, "Things are going well on the farm," you might write, "Bossy, that pretty blue-eyed cow you liked when you visited, just had twin calves." Or instead of saying, "I've mostly been going to a lot of movies," mention what movies and add a line or two about what you liked or disliked about them.

Sympathy Letters

Sometimes you will have to write a sympathy note. A friend's parent or grandparent may have died, or at some point you may even lose a friend and feel the need to write to the parents. Sympathy notes are admittedly difficult to write, but they mean so much to the person who receives them that you should not put off writing one when you know it will make someone feel better. And you should not send a card in place of a personal, hand-written note. You needn't say much. Here's an example:

Dear Mrs. Jones:
    I was so sorry to hear about the death of your mother.

I have a lovely memory of talking with her in the garden last summer when she visited you. She told me about the garden she remembered when she was a child and described so many of the flowers to me.

Please know that I am thinking of you in your time of loss.

Sincerely,
Becky

Sometimes you will be the one who has lost someone, and you will have to reply to a sympathy note. You need only write a brief note in response:

Dear Janet:

It was very kind of you to write and tell me such a lovely memory of Mother. I appreciate your thinking of me very much.

Fondly,
Sandy

Special Occasions

There will be occasions when you will want to send someone a greeting card—Mother's or Father's Day, birthdays, graduations, even some ethnic holidays or religious holidays are all good times to send cards. Choose a card carefully with the sender in mind, and think before you send an insulting or overly sarcastic card. You'll not be there to defend yourself against sensitive feelings when the card arrives.

Finally, and this is especially important for teens, don't write things in letters that you don't want others—especially parents or siblings—to read. You do live in a family, and while it is not polite to read another person's mail, it happens sometimes. The best way to avoid being embarrassed is not to put any of your secrets into writing.

Buying Gifts for Friends

You will on occasion want to buy a present either to celebrate a special friend or to celebrate a special occasion. The best rule of thumb about gift giving is never to give anything that will embarrass a friend—and this mostly has to do with money. Don't buy a present that is too expensive or that your friend could not afford to give in return. Most teens have a budget anyway, and clichéd as it sounds, it is the thought behind the gift that really matters. A little gift that shows a lot of thought is more meaningful than a big gift that was easily come by. (To learn about appropriate gifts to give boys, see Chapter 15.)

Overcoming Embarrassing Moments

Everyone has them, but somehow, when you're a teenager, embarrassing moments seem larger than life. You want to vanish, crawl under a chair, go up in a puff of smoke—certainly never again to go out with the boy that you just poured your soda all over. Don't worry about embarrassing moments. Keep in mind that you notice them far more than anyone around you does. Here are some specific hints on handling specific awkward situations:

Spilling Food or Drink. If you've spilled it on yourself, don't make a fuss. Wipe off as much of the food or beverage as you can, then excuse yourself to go to the ladies' room to finish the clean-up job. If you've spilled something on someone else, still don't make a big fuss. Say you are sorry. Hand the person a tissue, towel, or napkin to clean up with. And then be quiet. If something has obviously been spilled on a good outfit, say that you would like to pay for the dry cleaning. You will rarely be allowed to do so, but repeat the offer before dropping it.

Tearing an Outfit. If the rip is in an embarrassing place, you may find yourself in an especially awkward situation involving a little teasing. Simply smile, pick up your purse, which contains your emergency repair kit, and take yourself off to the ladies' room to make repairs.

Falling on the Dance Floor. Pick yourself up, make sure you aren't hurt, and continue dancing. If the person you are dancing with falls, show concern, ask him if he's alright, and if he wants to continue or sit down. Then do whatever he wants to do. Comment as little as possible on the situation.

Getting Your Period Unexpectedly. Despite the horror stories you have heard about girls who practically had to change high schools because of the Ultimate Embarrassment, you will rarely menstruate so heavily that blood will show on your clothes. If you do menstruate heavily, be prepared and extra-cautious. Change tampons or sanitary napkins frequently, and don't wear light-colored pants or skirts during your period. Be prepared and this will never happen to you.

Feeling Jealousy. Sometimes you see an old boyfriend with his new girlfriend, and the ugly green-eyed monster rears its head. Or sometimes you feel pangs over a friend's success and have trouble being as gracious as you might be.

Whatever the cause of your jealousy, pull yourself together and act gracious even if you do not feel that way. Greet your old boyfriend with a smile. If you are with someone, introduce him or her and be prepared to meet the person your former boyfriend is with. You needn't prolong your agony, however, and after saying hello and exchanging a few words, you can excuse yourself and move away.

When a friend has had some luck that you find hard to take (and who hasn't been in this situation at one time or another?), make an effort to be nice. Tell your friend how happy you are for her. If the luck or success is something really big—she made cheerleader and you didn't—and the friend is really close, you might want to discuss your feelings. Sometimes your first reaction is to pull away, and a friend wonders what she has done. If you feel yourself doing this, be big enough to call your friend, and say something like, "Judy, I want you to know that

I really am glad that you made cheerleader. As you might guess, I'm also sad that I didn't and maybe a little jealous, so if I act a little strange, I hope you will bear with me. I am happy for you." A gracious friend won't wave her successes in your face.

This chapter contains the basics for getting along with other people. There are also other places where you can turn for help. If you really feel a failure over your social relations, consider talking to a school counselor or therapist. If your problem is more specific, seek specific help. If you have a speech problem, for example, take some speech lessons. If you think your table manners lack a little polish, buy a book on table manners and read it.

Remember that manners are just a matter of making the other person feel at ease. Friendship is caring about others. Once you have mastered this, you will find that social success and wonderful friends pretty much fall into your lap.

17

THREE-WEEK MAKE-OVER PROGRAM

◄§ This chapter contains a three-week reducing diet and a three-week exercise program. There are also some suggestions for grooming and beauty rituals that you can use during this period.

We do not believe in make-overs that promise to turn you into a new person. For one thing, many teens are still experimenting to find out who they are, and they aren't quite ready to be given a new—and perhaps uncomfortable—look. Then, too, often people who appear so dramatically changed in magazine and newspaper make-overs do not maintain their "new" looks. We think your "look" should be one that you have developed over several months or years, and above all that it should be something you are completely at ease with. We do admit, though, that there are those times—the first of the year, just before bathing suit season, for example—when the urge to change overcomes us all. For those times, or any other time when you feel like giving yourself a lift, we suggest that you use the three-week diet and exercise program.

Feeling Fine Reducing Diet

In this diet, you are limited to approximately 1,700 calories per day—enough to meet your energy needs and still cause weight loss. While you should eat everything on the diet, you need not eat it in the order listed. This means, for example, that you can exchange a lunch and a dinner or that you can choose from any of the lunches listed for any day you want that meal.

There is nothing magical about this diet. It is based on consuming a reduced number of calories. The value of the diet lies in the structure it provides. You are told what to eat every day for twenty-one days, which eliminates a lot of time and thinking that you might spend planning a diet like this on your own. You should lose between 5 and 7 pounds.

While you are on this diet, you should take a one-a-day vitamin with iron and be sure to drink at least six glasses of water a day.

You may also find it helpful to reread Chapter 10 on dieting for any ideas and hints it provides.

Add a Dash of Creativity

The foods described here are fairly basic—what is left to your imagination is a variety of ways to make them more interesting.

You may, for example, add any spices and herbs you wish to these foods. A basic cookbook will contain a list of herbs and spices and the foods they go with; this should give you plenty of ideas. You can also use lemon juice, vinegar, a small amount of oil to mix with vinegar or lemon juice for salad dressing (although you will lose weight more quickly if you use only vinegar or lemon juice on salads), and small amounts of Worcestershire sauce. The Worcestershire is excellent on meats and also on grilled tomatoes.

Consider, too, using herbs and spices on the cooked vegetables; they are delicious and add a lot of flavor.

While dieting, do not use any steak sauce, but Worcestershire, catsup, or mustard, in small amounts, are okay. You may use very small amounts of mayonnaise where noted.

Breakfast
Eat this same breakfast every day for the diet.

tomato juice or ½ melon
egg, poached or boiled with 1
    teaspoon butter
1 slice toast, lightly buttered
skim milk, 8 ounces

Day 1

Lunch

egg salad sandwich on whole wheat bread
banana
skim milk, 8 ounces*

Dinner

whitefish, medium portion
green beans, ½ cup, cooked in water and salt
1 slice bread
butter, 1 teaspoon
milk
apple, medium

Day 2

Lunch

liverwurst sandwich on rye bread with light
    coating of mayonnaise
zucchini, ½ cup, cooked in water and salt
milk
peach

* all servings of milk are to be 8 ounces, skim

Dinner

ribeye steak, 3 ounces, broiled
spinach, ½ cup, cooked with water and salt
baked potato with 1 teaspoon butter
milk
pear

Day 3

Lunch

2 eggs, deviled
green beans, ½ cup, cooked in water and salt
milk
plums, 2 small

Dinner

chicken thigh, broiled, skin removed
broccoli, ½ cup, cooked in water and salt
tomato, baked or broiled
roll
butter, 1 teaspoon
milk
apple

Day 4

Lunch

flank steak, cold, broiled
rye bread, 2 slices, with light coating of butter
    or mayonnaise (make sandwich with steak)
tomato, sliced
milk
raisins, 1½-ounce box

Dinner

3-egg omelette made with mushrooms and green pepper
spinach, ½ cup, cooked with water and salt
asparagus, ½ cup, cooked with water and salt
milk
pear, medium

Day 5

Lunch

tuna salad sandwich on whole wheat bread
vegetable soup, 8 ounces
milk
banana

Dinner

lamb chops, 2 small, broiled
baked potato, medium
butter, 1 teaspoon
milk
plum

Day 6

Lunch

chef's salad, 3 cups (use lettuce and any other combination
  of salad vegetables you wish)
soft roll
butter, 1 teaspoon
milk
peach

Dinner

whitefish, medium portion
green beans, ½ cup, cooked in water and salt

tomato
1 slice bread
butter, 1 teaspoon
milk
plum, small

Day 7

Lunch

chicken breast, medium, broiled
zucchini, ½ cup, cooked in water and salt
vegetable soup, 8 ounces
soft roll
butter, 1 teaspoon
milk
plum, one small

Dinner

pot roast, made with 1 small potato, 1 tomato, 1 carrot,
    and beef boullion
soft roll
butter, 1 teaspoon
milk
melon, ½

Day 8

Lunch

liverwurst sandwich on rye bread
green beans and tomatoes, 1 cup
milk
apple

Dinner

whitefish, medium portion
asparagus, ½ cup, cooked in water and salt

baked potato
butter, 1 teaspoon
milk
peach

Day 9

Lunch

cottage cheese, ½ cup
tomato soup, 8 ounces
green beans, ½ cup, cooked in water and salt
soft roll
butter, 1 teaspoon
peach

Dinner

chicken leg and thigh, broiled, skin removed
broiled tomato
baked potato, small
butter, 1 teaspoon
milk
peach

Day 10

Lunch

tuna salad sandwich on whole wheat bread
tomato and cucumber, 1 cup
milk
banana

Dinner

hamburger, 3 ounces
rice, ½ cup
spinach, ½ cup, cooked in water and salt

small lettuce salad with ½ tomato
milk
apple

Day 11

Lunch

tuna salad sandwich on whole wheat bread
tomato soup, 8 ounces
green beans, ½ cup, cooked in water and salt
milk
apple

Dinner

whitefish, medium portion
rice, ½ cup
zucchini, ½ cup, cooked in water and salt
small lettuce salad
milk
plum, small

Day 12

Lunch

chicken thigh, broiled, skin removed
green beans, ½ cup, cooked in water and salt
sliced tomato, cucumber, and lettuce salad
milk
apple

Dinner

whitefish, medium portion
rice, ½ cup
zucchini and tomato, 1 cup, cooked in water and salt

asparagus, ½ cup, cooked in water and salt
milk
pear

Day 13

Lunch

chef's salad (lettuce, tomato, cucumber, carrot, and
    3 ounces ham or tongue)
soft roll
butter, 1 teaspoon
milk
peach

Dinner

ribeye steak, 3 ounces, broiled
spinach, ½ cup, cooked in water and salt
carrots, ½ cup, cooked in water and salt
baked potato
butter, 1 teaspoon
milk
plums, 2 medium

Day 14

Lunch

tuna salad sandwich on whole wheat bread
vegetable soup, 8 ounces
milk
apple

Dinner

whitefish, medium portion
green beans, ½ cup, cooked in salt and water
tomato, broiled

large lettuce salad with carrots and Spanish onions
milk
banana

Day 15

Lunch

2 eggs, deviled
cottage cheese, ½ cup
zucchini, 1 cup, cooked in water and salt
milk
apple, medium

Dinner

flank steak, 3 ounces, broiled
baked potato
tomato, broiled
asparagus, ½ cup, cooked in water and salt
butter, 1 teaspoon
milk
melon, ½

Day 16

Lunch

chicken breast, broiled, skin removed
green beans, ½ cup, cooked in water and salt
vegetable soup, 8 ounces
1 slice rye bread
butter, 1 teaspoon
milk
pear

Dinner

3-egg omelette with onions, mushrooms, and peppers
spinach, ½ cup

1 slice bread
butter, 1 teaspoon
milk
tangerine, small

Day 17

Lunch

egg salad sandwich on whole wheat bread
tomato soup, 8 ounces
milk
tangerine, small

Dinner

lamb chops, 2 small, broiled
green beans, ½ cup, cooked in water and salt
carrots, ½ cup, cooked in water and salt
small lettuce salad with ½ tomato
milk

Day 18

Lunch

liverwurst sandwich on rye bread
marinated tomato, cucumber, carrot, and onion salad
milk
banana

Dinner

shrimp, 10 medium, boiled and stir-fried with 1 tomato
    and 1 zucchini
green beans, ½ cup, cooked in water and salt
soft roll
butter, 1 teaspoon
milk
apple

Day 19

Lunch

hard cheese, 1 ounce
lettuce salad, 1 cup
roll
butter, 1 teaspoon
milk
banana

Dinner

whitefish, medium portion
carrots, ½ cup, cooked in water and salt
1 tomato and 1 zucchini, cooked together
roll
butter, 1 teaspoon
milk
apple

Day 20

Lunch

2 eggs, deviled
green beans, ½ cup, cooked in water and salt
tomato soup, 8 ounces
milk
tangerines, 2 medium

Dinner

chicken breast, broiled, skin removed
broccoli, ½ cup, cooked in water and salt
tomato, broiled
roll
butter, 1 teaspoon
milk
plums, 2 small

Day 21

Lunch

tuna salad sandwich on whole wheat bread
vegetable soup, 8 ounces
milk
raisins, 1½-ounce box

Dinner

whitefish, medium portion
green beans, ½ cup, cooked in water and salt
carrots, ½ cup, cooked in water and salt
lettuce salad, 1 cup
roll
butter, 1 teaspoon
milk
apple

EXERCISE PROGRAM

Exercise	Week 1		Week 2		Week 3	
	Days		*Days*		*Days*	
	1–3	4–7	1–3	4–7	1–3	4–7
Warm-Ups	full set	full set	full set	full set	full set	full set
Toe Touches	3	3	8	12	16	20
Lunges	4	4	6	6	8	10
Sit-Ups	5	5	8	10	12	15
Thigh Stretches		4	6	8	8	10
Leg Pulls		5	8	8	8	10
Leg Stretches			5	7	8	10
Leg Raises			4	7	8	10
Side Stretches			5	10	15	20
Push-Ups			2	4	6	6*
Balancer						1**

* Don't push on push-ups; you will be lucky if you can do 6. Just keep at them.

** This is a very difficult exercise. Keep trying until you master it.

Grooming Makeover

While you are improving yourself with diet and regular exercise, you may also want to reorganize your routine for daily and weekly grooming and take some special steps—such as a haircut—to add to your new look. Here are some suggestions.

Week 1

1. Write out a grooming program that you can follow with a minimum of time and effort and that will suit your and your family's time schedule.

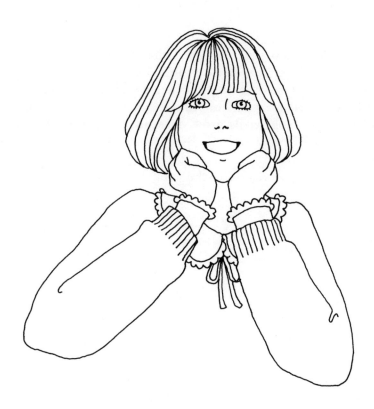

2. Draw up a list of supplies you will need.

3. Buy supplies

4. Experiment with any makeup you have bought.

5. Make a hair appointment if you need a new style or a shaping.

Week 2

1. Give yourself a facial or deep cleansing, whatever your skin type needs.

2. Give your hair a special conditioning or deep-oil treatment.

3. Give yourself a manicure but don't apply polish. Devote these two weeks to getting your nails and cuticles in good shape.

Week 3

1. Get a new hair style. Be sure to learn how to maintain it.

2. Clean and organize drawers and closets.

3. Try a facial mask or deep-cleanser treatment for your face.

4. Give yourself a manicure and apply polish; use clear if you are letting your nails grow out and a pretty light color if your nails are in good shape.

The new you is ready to face the public!

INDEX

INDEX